List of Contents

Introduction: The Awakening

Have you ever taken a moment to ponder the complexity of your relationship with food? In a world where it's all too easy to grab a quick bite on the go, to mindlessly munch on snacks while staring at screens, or to consume our emotions along with our meals, we've lost something profound along the way. We've lost our connection to food—our most basic and intimate connection to nature, to ourselves, and to the very essence of life.

Food isn't just sustenance; it's a powerful force that shapes our bodies, minds, and spirits. It's a source of nourishment, pleasure, and healing. It's a symbol of culture, tradition, and celebration. It's a reflection of our values, our emotions, and our innermost struggles. Food is life, and life is food. Yet, somewhere along the journey of modernity, we've allowed our most primal act—the act of eating—to become mundane, disconnected, and, for many, a source of profound confusion and suffering.

If you're reading this, it's likely that you've encountered your own battles with food and eating. Perhaps you've struggled with weight management, yo-yo dieting, or body image issues. Maybe you've fallen prey to the seductive allure of fast food, the mind-numbing comfort of emotional eating, or the endless cycle of restriction and indulgence. You're not alone. Millions of us share these struggles, navigating the labyrinthine landscape of our own eating habits, often with a mixture of frustration, guilt, and resignation.

But what if I told you that there's a path—a clear, practical, and deeply transformative path—that can liberate you from this cycle of suffering? What if I told you that you possess the innate power to reclaim your relationship with food, to rekindle your connection to your body, and to rediscover the joy of nourishment? This book is your invitation to embark on that journey—a journey into the heart of mindful eating.

In these pages, we won't dwell on dieting trends, calorie counting, or food restrictions. We won't engage in the tired battle of "good" versus "bad" foods, and we certainly won't prescribe a one-size-fits-all approach to eating. Instead, we'll dive deep into the profound wisdom of mindful eating—a practice that transcends diets, fads, and rigid rules. Mindful eating is not about perfection; it's about presence. It's not about deprivation; it's about choice. It's not about control; it's about liberation.

Now, you might wonder why I'm the one to guide you on this journey. Well, like many of you, I've walked the path of food-related struggles. I've grappled with body image issues, experimented with various diets, and fallen into the emotional eating trap. I know what it feels like to stand at the crossroads of self-doubt and self-acceptance, to yearn for a healthier relationship with food, and to search for a way out of the maze of mindless eating.

But here's what I've also learned: We don't have to be victims of our eating habits. We don't have to be held hostage by the diet industry or the relentless pressure to conform to unrealistic beauty standards. We have the power to reclaim our relationship with food, to break free from the cycle of guilt and restriction, and to savor the simple joys of nourishing our bodies and souls.

This book is the culmination of years of personal exploration, professional expertise, and the wisdom of countless individuals who have embarked on their own mindful eating journeys. It's not just a collection of theories and concepts; it's a practical roadmap for transformation. It's not about perfection; it's about progress. It's not about judgment; it's about self-compassion. It's not about deprivation; it's about abundance. It's not about rules; it's about mindful choices.

As we journey together through the chapters ahead, you'll discover that mindful eating isn't a rigid prescription but a flexible framework that adapts to your unique needs and circumstances. You'll learn that it's not about giving up your favorite foods but about savoring them with greater awareness. You'll realize that it's not about denying your emotions but about finding healthier ways to address them. Most importantly, you'll experience the profound freedom that comes from reconnecting with your body, your food, and your life.

Are you ready to embark on this transformative journey? Are you ready to awaken to the extraordinary power of mindful eating? If so, then let us begin. It's time to reclaim your relationship with food, nourish your body and soul, and rediscover the joy of truly living.

Chapter 1: Introduction to Mindful Eating

1.1 What is Mindful Eating?

In our fast-paced, modern world, where meals are often hurried affairs and food is readily available in abundance, the concept of mindful eating offers a refreshing and transformative approach to nourishing our bodies and souls. In this subchapter, we will delve into the essence of mindful eating, breaking it down into three fundamental aspects: Understanding the Basics, The Mind-Body Connection, and the myriad Benefits of Mindful Eating.

Understanding the Basics

Let's start at the beginning, shall we? Mindful eating isn't some esoteric concept reserved for meditation retreats and yoga studios. It's a fundamental approach to nourishing our bodies and souls, grounded in the simple act of paying attention.

At its core, mindful eating means being fully present during meals. It's about experiencing each bite with all your senses. It's the art of engaging in a deep, non-judgmental relationship with the food on your plate. In a world where we often inhale our meals while scrolling through our smartphones or zoning out in front of the TV, mindfulness at mealtime is like a lifeline to our well-being.

Picture this: You're seated at the dining table, your fork poised above a succulent piece of grilled asparagus. You take a moment to appreciate the vibrant green color, the slight char from the grill, and the earthy aroma. As you take that first bite, you're acutely aware of the tender crunch, the burst of flavor, and the nourishment it provides. You're not simply eating; you're experiencing, savoring, and truly living in that moment.

This isn't just about the asparagus, though. It's about every morsel you put in your mouth. Whether it's a juicy slice of watermelon on a scorching summer day or a hearty bowl of soup on a chilly evening, mindful eating invites you to show up, be present, and relish each mouthful.

The Mind-Body Connection
Now, here's where it gets fascinating. Mindful eating isn't just about tasting and savoring; it's also about tuning in to your body's cues and learning its language. You see, your body has an intricate network of hunger and fullness signals, much like a finely-tuned instrument waiting for you to listen.

Think about the last time you mindlessly devoured a bag of chips while binge-watching your favorite series. You probably didn't notice when you were comfortably full, did you? That's because you were disconnected from the messages your body was trying to send.

With mindful eating, you'll learn to decipher these signals. You'll understand the difference between true physical hunger and the emotional hunger that often leads to overeating. You'll become attuned to the gentle whispers of satisfaction and the subtle cues that tell you when it's time to put down your fork.

Imagine having the power to prevent overeating simply by listening to your body. Think of the freedom that comes from not obsessing over calorie counts or restrictive diets. That's the gift of the mind-body connection cultivated through mindful eating.

Benefits of Mindful Eating

So, why should you embark on this journey of mindful eating? What's in it for you, beyond the promise of a more harmonious relationship with food? The benefits are both profound and far-reaching.

1. Weight Management and Beyond: Let's address the elephant in the room - weight management. Mindful eating has shown its mettle in helping people shed excess pounds and maintain a healthy weight. When you eat mindfully, you're less likely to overindulge, and you're more attuned to your body's hunger and fullness cues. The result? A more balanced approach to weight management that doesn't involve drastic diets or deprivation.

2. Improved Relationship with Food: How often have you felt guilty after a so-called "cheat meal"? Mindful eating frees you from the shackles of guilt and shame. It encourages you to let go of the labels of "good" and "bad" foods and instead focus on the quality of your choices. Food is no longer your enemy but a source of nourishment and pleasure.

3. Emotional Well-being: Your relationship with food often mirrors your relationship with your emotions. Many of us turn to food for comfort, stress relief, or to numb difficult feelings. Mindful eating helps you break this cycle by offering healthier coping mechanisms. It invites you to explore the emotional landscape that drives your eating habits and provides tools to address those emotions in a constructive way.

4. Digestive Harmony: Digestion is a complex process influenced by both physical and mental factors. When you eat mindfully, you're more likely to chew your food thoroughly, aiding the digestive process. Additionally, the reduction of stress and anxiety around eating can alleviate digestive issues like bloating and indigestion.

5. Enhanced Taste Sensations: Ever noticed how a simple piece of fruit can taste like an explosion of flavors when you're truly present? Mindful eating elevates your sensory experience, allowing you to relish the nuances and subtleties of different foods. Suddenly, everyday meals become a feast for your senses.

6. Stress Reduction: In our fast-paced world, mealtime is often a hurried affair. Mindful eating provides a respite from the chaos. By slowing down and savoring your meals, you create a mini oasis of calm in your day. This can have a ripple effect, reducing overall stress levels and improving your overall well-being.

So, there you have it—mindful eating in a nutshell. It's the antithesis to the mindless munching that has become all too common in our lives. It's a gateway to a healthier, more conscious relationship with food, your body, and yourself. As we journey through the chapters of this book, you'll learn not just what mindful eating is but how to weave it into the fabric of your daily life, making it a natural and empowering part of your wellness routine. So, let's dive in and uncover the transformative power of mindful eating together.

1.2 The Ideal Body Myth

In the pursuit of health and wellness, we often find ourselves entangled in the web of societal ideals. It's a trap we all fall into at one point or another—the belief that there exists a singular, elusive "ideal body." This belief, this myth, has a way of creeping into our minds, infiltrating our thoughts, and dictating our actions. It's as if we're chasing a phantom, an illusion, and we do so at the risk of losing our sense of self, our authenticity, and our inner peace.

But here's the truth, and it's a truth I've learned through years of research, introspection, and working with countless individuals seeking a healthier relationship with food and their bodies: the ideal body is a myth, a mirage on the horizon, forever out of reach.

Debunking Unrealistic Expectations

Society's portrayal of the "ideal body" is a constantly shifting target, a chameleon that adapts to the whims of fashion and media. What's deemed ideal today may be obsolete tomorrow. It's an ever-changing landscape of unattainable standards that leaves us perpetually dissatisfied, chasing an image of beauty that's as fleeting as it is unattainable.

Consider the images that bombard us daily—Photoshopped models on magazine covers, meticulously curated social media feeds, and advertisements promising miraculous transformations with the latest fad diet or exercise gadget. These images often showcase a version of reality that's far removed from the truth. Behind the scenes, there are teams of makeup artists, photographers, and digital wizards manipulating every pixel, erasing blemishes, nipping and tucking, until the final product bears little resemblance to the person in the photo.

This unattainable ideal is the root of much of our frustration and self-doubt. We end up feeling inadequate, as if we don't measure up to an impossible standard. The pursuit of such a mirage can lead to a cycle of self-loathing, crash diets, and unsustainable exercise regimens—all in the name of attaining the unattainable.

But I want you to understand something essential: **you are not meant to conform to these unrealistic expectations**. Your worth is not determined by your appearance. The beauty industry thrives on our insecurities, perpetuating the myth that we need to be fixed. In reality, we are not broken. It is the standards that are broken. It's time to break free from this cycle of self-critique and realize that you are enough, just as you are.

The Importance of Healthy Goals

In our journey towards mindful eating and a healthier relationship with our bodies, it's crucial to redefine our goals. Rather than fixating on the elusive ideal body, let's shift our focus to something more profound—health and well-being.

Consider this: What if, instead of striving for a particular number on the scale or a dress size, you aimed to feel vibrant, energetic, and truly alive? What if you aspired to nourish your body with foods that made you thrive, to move in ways that brought joy, and to cultivate a sense of inner peace and self-acceptance?

This shift in perspective can be truly transformative. It's about setting goals that prioritize your well-being, both physically and mentally. It's about choosing foods that nourish you, rather than depriving yourself. It's about engaging in physical activity that you enjoy, rather than punishing yourself through grueling workouts. It's about embracing a positive relationship with your body, free from the toxic influence of external standards.

Consider this a moment of empowerment. Your health is not defined by your appearance but by how you feel, how well your body functions, and your overall sense of vitality. Healthy goals are about finding balance, not extremes. They're about creating a lifestyle that's sustainable and enjoyable, not about quick fixes or deprivation.

Embracing Body Positivity

One of the most powerful tools in our journey towards mindful eating is the concept of body positivity. At its core, body positivity is a revolutionary act of self-love and acceptance. It's about rejecting the notion that your worth is tied to your appearance and recognizing that your body is incredible just as it is, with all its uniqueness and imperfections.

We live in a world that often teaches us to be critical of ourselves, to scrutinize every inch of our bodies, and to fixate on our flaws. Body positivity is a counter-narrative to this destructive mindset. It encourages us to celebrate our bodies for what they do rather than how they look.

Embracing body positivity means acknowledging that your body is your lifelong companion, carrying you through every experience, every challenge, and every joy in life. It's the vessel that allows you to explore the world, connect with others, and savor the simple pleasures of existence. Your body is not your enemy; it's your ally on this journey of life.

Let's be clear—body positivity doesn't mean that you have to be in love with every aspect of your body every single day. It's about practicing self-compassion and accepting that it's okay to have moments of doubt or insecurity. It's about challenging negative self-talk and actively working to replace it with self-affirming thoughts.

Body positivity is not a destination; it's a practice—a daily commitment to treating yourself with kindness, respect, and love. It's about embracing the idea that you are worthy of love and care, regardless of your size, shape, or appearance.

The journey we're embarking upon is a profound one—a journey towards mindful eating and a healthier, more compassionate relationship with our bodies. It begins with understanding that the ideal body is a myth, one that we need not chase. Instead, we can redefine our goals, focusing on health and well-being, and we can embrace body positivity, learning to love and celebrate the incredible vessel that is our body. This is a journey of empowerment, self-acceptance, and transformation—one that you are more than capable of undertaking.

1.3 How Mindful Eating Can Transform Your Life

Mindful eating is more than just a practice; it's a path to transformation. In the following pages, we will delve into the profound ways in which mindful eating can reshape your life, from your relationship with your body to your emotional well-being. While weight management is often the initial motivator for many, mindful eating transcends the scale, offering a holistic approach to nourishing both body and soul.

Weight Management and Beyond

When we first hear about mindful eating, it's not uncommon for our thoughts to gravitate towards weight management. In a world obsessed with body image and quick-fix diets, it's easy to see why. However, mindful eating isn't just another diet; it's a sustainable way of life that, over time, can lead to a healthier weight without the rollercoaster of deprivation and guilt.

The secret of mindful eating lies in awareness. It's about being present in the moment, understanding your body's cues, and making conscious choices. When you eat mindfully, you become attuned to your body's hunger and fullness signals. No more overeating until you're uncomfortably stuffed, or mindless snacking out of boredom. Instead, you'll eat when you're hungry and stop when you're satisfied.

The act of savoring each bite, truly tasting the flavors, and experiencing the textures is a game-changer. It slows down your eating pace, allowing your body the time it needs to register fullness. Over time, this simple shift in behavior can lead to weight loss or maintenance without the need for strict diets or calorie counting.

But the transformative power of mindful eating extends beyond the physical realm. It's about fostering a harmonious relationship with food, one that frees you from the clutches of guilt and obsession. It's about finding balance, making peace with your plate, and appreciating the nourishment it provides. It's an invitation to let go of the cycle of dieting and embrace a lifestyle that allows you to relish food without regrets.

Improved Relationship with Food

Our relationship with food is often deeply intertwined with our emotions. We celebrate with food, seek comfort in it, and sometimes use it to fill emotional voids. Mindful eating sheds light on this complex connection, offering us a chance to untangle our emotions from our eating habits.

When you eat mindfully, you become aware of emotional triggers that lead to overeating or unhealthy food choices. You begin to recognize the difference between physical hunger and emotional hunger. Instead of reaching for a bag of chips when you're stressed or lonely, you pause and ask yourself, "Am I truly hungry, or am I seeking comfort?"

This newfound awareness empowers you to respond to emotional hunger in healthier ways. You might opt for a walk, call a friend, or engage in a creative activity to soothe your emotions instead of turning to food. It's a transformation that goes beyond what's on your plate; it's a transformation of your emotional well-being.

Moreover, as you practice mindful eating, you start to appreciate the taste of food on a whole new level. The vibrant colors of fresh produce, the aroma of herbs and spices, the intricate blend of flavors in a well-prepared meal – all of these become sources of joy. Food ceases to be a mere means of sustenance; it becomes an experience to savor and celebrate.

Emotional Well-being

Now, let's talk about perhaps the most profound transformation that mindful eating can bring into your life: emotional well-being. Our emotions are intricately linked to our eating habits. How many times have you turned to food to alleviate stress, anxiety, or sadness? In these moments, food becomes a crutch, a way to numb or distract from uncomfortable emotions.

Mindful eating doesn't just teach you to eat with awareness; it helps you navigate the complex terrain of your emotions. It encourages you to recognize emotional eating patterns and to respond with compassion. When you're feeling overwhelmed, instead of reaching for a bag of chips, you learn to pause and ask yourself, "What am I truly feeling right now?" This pause is powerful; it creates a space for self-reflection and self-care.

Emotional eating is often an attempt to fill an emotional void. Mindful eating invites you to explore healthier ways of coping with emotions, such as journaling, meditation, or talking to a trusted friend or therapist. It's about acknowledging that food can't heal emotional wounds but that self-compassion and self-care can.

With mindful eating, you'll discover that you have the capacity to sit with your emotions, to acknowledge them without judgment, and to make choices that honor your well-being. You'll find that food loses its grip as your primary source of comfort, and you'll develop a deeper connection with yourself and your emotional landscape.

Mindful eating offers you the tools to transform your relationship with food, your body, and your emotions. It's a journey of self-discovery and self-compassion, a path to sustainable weight management, and a gateway to emotional well-being. As we continue this exploration, we'll delve deeper into the practical aspects of mindful eating and provide you with actionable steps to embark on this transformative journey. The power to change your life through mindful eating is within your grasp, and it starts with a simple choice: to be present with your food and with yourself.

Chapter 2: The Science of Mindful Eating

2.1 The Psychology Behind Mindful Eating

In our relentless pursuit of health and happiness, we often find ourselves at odds with the very act that sustains us: eating. We shovel down our meals in a hurry, barely taking the time to register the flavors or textures. Our minds are elsewhere—engrossed in work, consumed by worries, or distracted by the ceaseless chatter of our digital devices. In this frantic pace of modern life, eating has become a mundane and mechanical task, devoid of its natural grace.

But what if I told you that within this seemingly mundane act lies the key to a profound transformation in your relationship with food, your body, and your overall well-being? Welcome to the world of mindful eating, where every bite is an opportunity for self-discovery and self-care.

Awareness of Eating Habits

The journey into mindful eating begins with a fundamental shift: the awakening of awareness. It's about recognizing that the way you eat is as important as what you eat. Our eating habits are deeply ingrained, often developed over a lifetime, and largely influenced by external factors like family, culture, and society. We tend to operate on autopilot, unaware of the choices we make and the impact they have on our bodies.

Becoming aware of your eating habits is like switching on a light in a dimly lit room. Suddenly, you can see the patterns, the triggers, and the emotions that govern your relationship with food. This newfound awareness empowers you to make conscious choices rather than succumbing to mindless impulses.

Imagine this scenario: You've had a long and stressful day at work. You arrive home exhausted, and the first thing you do is head to the kitchen. Before you know it, you've polished off a bag of chips while standing at the counter, barely tasting a morsel. Sound familiar? That's mindless eating at its finest—a reaction to stress, habit, or simply a lack of awareness.

When you introduce mindfulness into this equation, everything changes. You pause before reaching for that bag of chips. You take a deep breath and ask yourself, "Am I truly hungry, or am I eating out of habit or stress?" This simple pause creates a space for choice. You might decide to have a small, mindful snack or opt for a relaxing cup of tea instead. This awareness transforms eating from an automatic reaction into a conscious decision, giving you control over your choices.

Breaking the Cycle of Emotional Eating
Emotions and eating are often deeply entangled. From celebrating with a slice of cake to drowning sorrows in a tub of ice cream, food becomes a comforting ally during emotional storms. This, my friends, is emotional eating, and it's a cycle that many of us are caught in.

Mindful eating equips us with the tools to break this cycle. By bringing mindfulness to our emotional states, we learn to differentiate between true hunger and emotional hunger. We discover that there are better ways to cope with our feelings than through food alone.

Picture this scenario: After a tough day at work, you find yourself reaching for a bag of cookies. But with mindful awareness, you take a breath and ask yourself, "What am I really feeling right now?" You may realize it's not hunger but stress or frustration. In that moment, you've disrupted the emotional eating cycle.

Mindful vs. Mindless Eating
Perhaps you're wondering what distinguishes mindful eating from its mindless counterpart. The difference lies not only in the act itself but in the profound impact it has on your well-being.

Mindless eating is like a mechanical dance with food. You chew, swallow, and repeat, hardly noticing the flavors or textures. Your mind drifts elsewhere, and before you know it, the meal is over, leaving you unsatisfied and disconnected from your body's signals.

Mindful eating, on the other hand, is a sensory experience. It's about engaging all your senses—sight, smell, touch, taste, and even sound—in the act of eating. It's like savoring a symphony of flavors with each bite, truly relishing the culinary masterpiece before you.

Imagine this: You're sitting down to a meal of sushi—a delicacy renowned for its intricate flavors and textures. As you pick up a piece of sushi with your chopsticks, you take a moment to observe its presentation—the vibrant colors, the artful arrangement, and the glistening rice. You inhale deeply, savoring the aroma of the freshly prepared ingredients.

With mindful intention, you bring the sushi to your mouth, feeling the coolness of the rice and the subtle resistance of the nori seaweed. As you take a bite, you let the flavors dance on your taste buds—the sweet tang of pickled ginger, the umami richness of soy sauce, and the delicate freshness of the fish.

In this moment of mindful eating, you are fully present, immersed in the culinary experience. Your senses are heightened, and the simple act of eating becomes a celebration of life. You eat slowly, savoring each bite, and you stop when you feel satisfied, not when the plate is empty.

This, my dear readers, is the essence of mindful eating—a profound shift from mechanical consumption to a sensory celebration of food. It's a journey that invites you to embrace the fullness of the present moment, to connect with your body's wisdom, and to nourish yourself on a deeper level than ever before.

2.2 The Physiology of Mindful Eating

In the quest for a healthier, more balanced life, it's essential to delve into the science behind mindful eating. The way our bodies react to what we eat is a key piece of the mindful eating puzzle. By understanding the physiological processes at play, you can unlock the potential of this transformative practice to reshape your relationship with food and, subsequently, your overall well-being.

Digestion and Metabolism

Let's begin our exploration with digestion and metabolism, two fundamental aspects that the practice of mindful eating can significantly influence. You see, it's not just about what you eat but how you eat it.

Digestion is a marvel of the human body, a complex dance of enzymes, acids, and muscular contractions. When you eat mindlessly, hurriedly gobbling down your meal without paying attention, you disrupt this finely tuned process. The body struggles to keep up, leading to discomfort, indigestion, and even the dreaded food coma.

However, when you practice mindful eating, something extraordinary happens. By slowing down and savoring each bite, you give your digestive system the time it needs to shine. Chewing your food thoroughly, you begin the digestive process in your mouth, breaking down carbohydrates and initiating the release of digestive enzymes. With each chew, you're sending a signal to your stomach: "Hey, get ready, food's on the way!"

As you continue to eat mindfully, your body responds in kind. The stomach releases gastric juices in an orderly fashion, promoting efficient digestion. The nutrients from your food are absorbed more effectively, providing your body with the fuel it needs to thrive.

But it doesn't stop there. Mindful eating goes even further by influencing your metabolism. When you're truly present with your meal, you allow your body to better regulate its energy expenditure. You're less likely to overeat, which means fewer excess calories that your body would have to store as fat. Instead, you supply your body with the right amount of energy it requires.

Mindful eating helps you become in sync with your body's natural rhythms, enhancing both digestion and metabolism. It's not a magic pill for weight loss, but rather a sustainable approach to nourishing your body optimally.

Mindful Eating and Hormonal Balance
Now, let's journey into the fascinating world of hormones, those tiny chemical messengers that wield incredible power over your body. In the context of mindful eating, hormones play a critical role in controlling your appetite, regulating your weight, and influencing your mood.

One of the key hormones at play here is leptin. Think of leptin as your body's hunger meter. It's produced by your fat cells and signals to your brain that you're full. However, chronic overeating, especially when it's rushed and mindless, can lead to a condition known as leptin resistance. Your brain becomes desensitized to leptin's signals, and you end up feeling hungry even when you've had enough to eat.

This is where mindful eating comes to the rescue. When you eat slowly and savor each bite, your body has more time to release leptin and signal fullness effectively. It's like tuning up your hunger meter, making it more accurate and responsive.

Additionally, mindful eating helps balance another hormone called ghrelin, often dubbed the hunger hormone. Ghrelin stimulates your appetite, and its levels typically rise before meals. However, when you're rushing through meals or snacking mindlessly, ghrelin can remain elevated, leading to constant cravings.

By practicing mindfulness during meals, you can better regulate ghrelin production. As you become more attuned to your body's hunger cues, you'll notice that ghrelin's cries for food become more aligned with your actual needs.

Nutrient Absorption
Finally, let's explore the crucial topic of nutrient absorption—a cornerstone of our health that's often overlooked in the rush of modern life. Your body requires an array of vitamins, minerals, and other nutrients to function optimally. However, merely ingesting these nutrients isn't enough; they must be effectively absorbed into your bloodstream to benefit your body.

Enter mindful eating. When you engage in this practice, you're not just enhancing digestion and hormonal balance; you're also increasing the efficiency of nutrient absorption.

Consider the role of enzymes in breaking down food. These specialized proteins are essential for nutrient absorption. When you're rushed or stressed while eating, enzyme production can be compromised. This means your body may struggle to extract all the valuable nutrients from your food.

In contrast, when you approach your meal with mindfulness, you create an environment conducive to proper enzyme secretion. Your body recognizes that it's time to digest, and it responds accordingly. As a result, you're better equipped to absorb the vitamins and minerals that are essential for vitality and well-being.

Moreover, mindfulness extends beyond the act of eating itself. It can influence your food choices, leading you to select nutrient-dense, whole foods rather than highly processed, nutrient-poor options. By choosing foods rich in vitamins, minerals, and antioxidants, you're providing your body with the raw materials it needs for optimal function.

Mindful eating is like a key that unlocks the treasure trove of nutrients in your food. It ensures that the nourishment you consume is not wasted but utilized to its fullest extent, supporting your overall health and vitality.

As you can see, the physiology of mindful eating is a remarkable journey into the inner workings of your body.

By practicing mindfulness at the table, you're not only nurturing your physical health but also cultivating a deeper connection with your body's wisdom. This is the foundation upon which your path to lasting well-being is built, one mindful bite at a time.

2.3 Mindful Eating and Longevity

In the quest for a longer and healthier life, the age-old adage "you are what you eat" holds an undeniable truth. While the connection between food and longevity is not a newfound revelation, the art of mindful eating is transforming how we approach our dietary choices and, in turn, our prospects for a longer and more vibrant life.

Reducing the Risk of Chronic Diseases

In the modern age of convenience and fast-paced living, chronic diseases have surged to the forefront of our health concerns. Heart disease, diabetes, hypertension, and various cancers have become all too common in our society. But what if I told you that the power to reduce your risk of these chronic diseases lies in the very act of how you eat your meals?

Mindful eating isn't merely a fleeting trend; it's a scientifically-backed approach to health and longevity. Research has consistently shown that individuals who embrace mindful eating practices are at a significantly lower risk of developing chronic diseases. Why? Because they're not only attentive to what they eat but how they eat it.

Picture this: a person who practices mindful eating sits down to enjoy a meal. They savor each bite, fully engaging with the colors, textures, and flavors on their plate. They listen to their body's hunger cues, knowing precisely when to stop eating. This level of awareness ensures that they make healthier food choices, consume appropriate portion sizes, and, over time, lower their risk of chronic diseases.

Furthermore, mindful eating encourages the consumption of whole, nutrient-dense foods—those that are rich in antioxidants, vitamins, and minerals. These foods act as a protective shield for your body, combating inflammation and oxidative stress, two factors that play a pivotal role in the development of chronic diseases. So, it's not just about what you're avoiding but also about what you're embracing on your plate.

As you embrace mindful eating as a way of life, you're not just making a temporary change in your diet; you're making a profound investment in your long-term health and longevity.

Enhancing Cellular Health
The inner workings of our bodies are nothing short of astonishing. Our trillions of cells operate like tiny machines, performing tasks that keep us alive and functioning optimally. The health of our cells is, in many ways, a reflection of the health of our overall body. And

guess what? Mindful eating has the power to optimize the very core of our existence—our cells.

Our cells are under constant attack from oxidative stress and inflammation. These threats can cause cellular damage, premature aging, and even lead to the development of chronic diseases. However, mindful eating can be our ally in the fight against these internal assailants.

When we consume meals mindfully, we're making choices that provide our cells with the essential nutrients they need to thrive. Antioxidants, for instance, found in fruits, vegetables, and whole grains, act as bodyguards for our cells, neutralizing harmful free radicals and preventing cellular damage. Essential vitamins and minerals play crucial roles in cellular functions, from energy production to DNA repair.

Furthermore, mindful eating promotes a balanced and stable blood sugar level. This helps prevent insulin spikes and crashes, which can damage cells over time. When you savor each bite and choose foods that release energy slowly, you're providing your cells with a consistent source of fuel, enhancing their longevity and vitality.

Moreover, the stress-reduction aspect of mindful eating is vital in promoting cellular health. Chronic stress takes a toll on our cells, speeding up the aging process and leaving us vulnerable to diseases. Mindful eating practices like deep breathing and relaxation before meals can lower stress hormones, creating an internal environment that supports cellular well-being.

Every bite you take, every mindful meal you enjoy, is a step towards enhancing the health and longevity of your cells. You're not just eating; you're nurturing the very essence of your being.

Long-term Health Benefits

Now, let's delve into the long-term health benefits of mindful eating, because the true power of this practice lies not only in the present but also in the years and decades that lie ahead.

Imagine a life free from the constant battle of yo-yo dieting, weight fluctuations, and the rollercoaster of fad diets. Mindful eating provides you with a sustainable and practical approach to maintaining a healthy weight throughout your life. By listening to your body's hunger and fullness cues, you naturally regulate your food intake. This means no more cycles of deprivation followed by overindulgence—just a steady, balanced way of eating that supports your well-being.

As you age, the importance of bone health becomes increasingly evident. Osteoporosis and fractures become genuine concerns. Thankfully, mindful eating doesn't just focus on the quantity of food you eat but also on the quality. Calcium-rich foods like leafy greens, fortified plant-based milk, and almonds can be integral components of your mindful eating plan. These foods contribute to strong and resilient bones, ensuring you enjoy a vibrant life well into your golden years.

Furthermore, mindful eating supports heart health, reducing the risk of cardiovascular diseases. By making heart-healthy choices—opting for plant-based oils, whole grains, and plenty of fruits and vegetables—you're actively working to maintain a robust cardiovascular system. Plus, the stress-reduction element of mindful eating helps maintain healthy blood pressure levels, which is a significant factor in heart health.

The longevity-enhancing effects of mindful eating extend to brain health as well. Studies have shown that a diet rich in antioxidants, omega-3 fatty acids, and other brain-boosting nutrients can slow cognitive decline and reduce the risk of neurodegenerative diseases like Alzheimer's. And guess what? These are precisely the types of foods that are often emphasized in mindful eating.

Mindful eating isn't just about living longer; it's about living better. It's about embracing each moment with vitality and grace. It's about savoring the flavors of your journey and nourishing your body in a way that allows it to thrive. It's about reducing the risk of chronic diseases, enhancing cellular health, and reaping the long-term benefits of a practice that's as timeless as it is powerful.

Incorporating mindful eating into your daily life isn't just a temporary fix; it's a lifelong commitment to your well-being. It's an investment in the years ahead, each bite and each moment adding to the richness of your journey. So, embrace mindful eating not just for today, but for the tomorrows that await, filled with health, vitality, and the gift of longevity.

Chapter 3: Building a Mindful Eating Foundation

3.1 Cultivating Mindfulness

In the quest for a revolutionary transformation in our relationship with food, mindfulness becomes our most potent ally. It's the cornerstone upon which our mindful eating foundation is built. Through the lens of mindfulness, we learn to savor every bite, to appreciate the symphony of flavors and textures, and to listen closely to our body's signals. This chapter delves deep into the heart of cultivating mindfulness in our daily lives, offering practical techniques that will pave the way for mindful eating to flourish.

Mindful Meditation Practices

Meditation is the art of turning inward, a practice that has been honed for centuries to cultivate a profound sense of presence and awareness. As you embark on your journey towards mindful eating, consider meditation as your silent companion, guiding you through the labyrinth of your mind and emotions.

Mindful Meditation: A Personal Sanctuary

Picture this: You find a quiet spot, a place where you won't be disturbed. You sit comfortably, your spine erect but not rigid, your hands resting gently on your lap. You close your eyes, and for the first time in a long while, you truly listen—to your breath. The inhale, the exhale, the rise and fall of your chest. This is where your mindful meditation begins.

The purpose of mindful meditation is not to empty your mind but to observe it without judgment. As thoughts bubble to the surface like pebbles in a clear stream, you don't push them away; you simply acknowledge their presence and let them drift away. Your breath becomes your anchor, grounding you in the present moment.

As you continue this practice, you'll notice something extraordinary: the ability to separate yourself from your thoughts and emotions. You'll realize that you are not your cravings, your anxieties, or your desires. You are the observer, the witness to your inner world.

Mindful meditation is not a quick fix; it's a journey. Each session is a step toward a more profound connection with your inner self. Over time, you'll find that the stillness you cultivate in meditation begins to infuse other aspects of your life, especially your eating habits.

The Ripple Effect of Mindful Meditation

The ripple effect of mindful meditation extends far beyond the moments you spend on the cushion. It gradually seeps into your everyday life. You become more attuned to your body's signals, more aware of the choices you make, and more in control of your reactions.

When faced with a tempting snack, you'll pause. Instead of impulsively reaching for it, you'll take a moment to check in with your body. Are you truly hungry, or is it just a passing craving? You'll notice the sensations in your stomach—the gentle rumbling, the subtle cues. And in that pause, that brief moment of mindfulness, you'll find the power to make a conscious choice.

Mindful meditation is your training ground, your sanctuary. It's where you strengthen the muscle of awareness, the core element of mindful eating. Embrace it with patience and consistency, and watch it transform your relationship with food.

Mindful Breathing Techniques
Breath—the most primal and vital of human functions. It is both an involuntary and voluntary act, a bridge between our conscious and unconscious worlds. In the realm of mindful eating, harnessing the power of your breath can be a game-changer.

The Breath as an Anchor

In the chaos of our modern lives, we often forget the simple beauty of breathing. It's always with us, yet we rarely pay it any heed. But in the practice of mindful eating, your breath can become an anchor, a lifeline to the present moment.

Begin by taking a moment to observe your breath. Feel the air entering your nostrils, cool and refreshing. Follow it as it fills your lungs, expanding your chest and belly. Then, as you exhale, notice the warmth and the release. This is the rhythm of life itself—the inhale, the exhale, a continuous cycle.

As you sit down to a meal, bring your attention to your breath. Take a few deep breaths, inhaling slowly through your nose and exhaling gently through your mouth. Let your breath settle into a natural, unforced rhythm.

Breath and Mindful Eating

Now, let's connect the dots between your breath and your eating habits. Imagine a scenario: you're at a restaurant, and a plate of your favorite pasta is placed before you. The aroma wafts up, and your mouth waters. Before diving in, take a breath.

Inhale deeply, savoring the scent, and exhale slowly. This simple act creates a pause, a moment of mindfulness. It allows you to acknowledge your excitement, your anticipation, without judgment. It allows you to be fully present as you lift your fork, twirl the pasta, and take that first bite.

As you chew, continue to breathe consciously. Feel the texture of the food, the flavors unfolding on your palate. Notice how your body responds to each bite. Your breath keeps you grounded in the experience, preventing you from rushing through the meal.

The Power of Pauses

Mindful breathing isn't just about the breath itself; it's about the pauses it creates. These pauses are where the magic happens. They're the moments when you reconnect with your body, your senses, and your true hunger.

Before reaching for that second helping, take a breath. Pause and ask yourself, "Am I still hungry? Do I truly want more?" This pause allows you to differentiate between physical hunger and the desire to continue eating out of habit or emotion.

Mindful breathing techniques are your allies in creating those essential pauses. They remind you to slow down, to savor, and to listen to your body's cues. Over time, they become second nature, woven into the fabric of your mindful eating practice.

Creating Mindful Habits

Habits, those automatic routines deeply ingrained in our lives, can be our greatest allies or our most formidable adversaries when it comes to mindful eating. But the good news is that habits are malleable, adaptable, and subject to change. By harnessing the power of mindfulness, you can transform your habits and, in turn, your relationship with food.

The Habit Loop

Habits operate on a simple yet powerful loop: cue, routine, reward. Let's take the example of mindless snacking in front of the television. The cue might be boredom or stress, the routine is reaching for a bag of chips, and the reward is the momentary distraction and the salty crunch.

To transform this habit, we introduce mindfulness into the equation. As soon as you recognize the cue—boredom or stress—take a mindful pause. Close your eyes, take a few deep breaths, and tune into the emotions or sensations you're experiencing. This is your opportunity to choose a new routine, a mindful one.

The Power of Intention

Creating mindful habits begins with intention. It's about making a conscious decision to change your automatic responses. But intention alone isn't enough; you need a clear plan.

Let's say you want to incorporate mindful eating into your lunchtime routine at work. First, set a clear intention: "I intend to eat my lunch mindfully every day this week." Next, create a plan: "I will turn off all electronic devices, find a quiet spot, and eat slowly, savoring each bite."

Start Small, Think Big

Remember, creating mindful habits is a gradual process. Start small, focusing on one habit at a time. Maybe it's mindfully drinking a glass of water each morning or pausing for a deep breath before a snack. Once you've mastered one habit, move on to the next.

As you nurture these mindful habits, you'll find that they begin to shape your daily life. They become the foundation upon which your mindful eating practice thrives. Over time, you'll observe a profound shift in your relationship with food, one grounded in awareness, choice, and intention.

Cultivating mindfulness is not a sprint; it's a marathon—a lifelong journey. It's a path filled with moments of stillness, breath, and conscious choice. It's a journey that will transform not only the way you eat but also the way you experience life.

So, embrace these practices with an open heart and a curious mind. Approach them not as chores but as gifts you give to yourself—a roadmap to a life of greater awareness, fulfillment, and the ideal body you deserve.

3.2 Mindful Food Choices

In our journey towards mindful eating, the foundation upon which we build our relationship with food is pivotal. It's here, in the realm of mindful food choices, that we learn to navigate the labyrinth of supermarket aisles and restaurant menus with intention and awareness. By making conscious decisions about what we eat, we not only nourish our bodies but also contribute to a healthier planet and a more sustainable food system. In this subchapter, we delve into the art of mindful food choices, exploring how understanding food labels, opting for whole and nutrient-dense foods, and embracing local and sustainable options can empower us on our path to mindful eating mastery.

Understanding Food Labels

In our fast-paced world, food labels have become our trusted companions in the grocery store aisles. They are the cryptic codes that unveil the mysteries of what lies within those neatly packaged boxes and cans. However, deciphering these labels can sometimes feel like deciphering a foreign language. What do those numbers and percentages really mean, and how do they impact our mindful eating journey?

Let's demystify the art of reading food labels. Begin by scanning the ingredient list—the heart and soul of any packaged product. Here, the most abundant ingredients are listed first. A mindful eater looks for simplicity in this list, favoring products with recognizable, whole-food ingredients. If a label reads like a chemistry experiment, it might be time to reconsider your choice.

Next, focus on the serving size. Many people overlook this crucial detail, which can lead to overeating without even realizing it. Be mindful of portion sizes, and remember that the nutritional information provided is based on one serving. To get an accurate understanding of what you're consuming, do the math if you plan to eat more or less than the recommended serving size.

Now, let's explore the nutritional panel, which provides insight into calories, macronutrients (like fats, proteins, and carbohydrates), and micronutrients (like vitamins and minerals). While these numbers are essential, a mindful eater approaches them with balance in mind. Rather than obsessing over calorie counts or macronutrient ratios, focus on the overall quality of the food. Is it nutrient-dense? Does it provide valuable vitamins and minerals? Does it align with your personal health goals? These questions guide us toward making informed food choices.

Choosing Whole and Nutrient-Dense Foods

In the world of mindful eating, the spotlight shines brightly on whole and nutrient-dense foods. These culinary heroes are the ones that nourish our bodies, providing the essential nutrients required for optimal health. But what exactly are whole and nutrient-dense foods, and how do they fit into our daily lives?

Whole foods are, simply put, foods that are as close to their natural state as possible. They are unprocessed or minimally processed and are free from additives, preservatives, and artificial flavors. Think of vibrant fruits and vegetables, whole grains like brown rice and quinoa, lean proteins such as chicken or tofu, and nuts and seeds. These foods are rich in vitamins, minerals, fiber, and antioxidants—nutritional powerhouses that support our well-being.

Nutrient-dense foods, on the other hand, are foods that pack a nutritional punch per calorie. They are high in nutrients relative to their calorie content, making them an excellent choice for mindful eaters. Leafy greens, berries, beans, and fish are prime examples. Incorporating these foods into your diet can help you meet your nutritional needs without overloading on calories.

But how do we make whole and nutrient-dense foods a central part of our diets? Start by shifting your perspective on meal planning. Instead of focusing on what you need to exclude from your meals, concentrate on what you can add. Build your plate around colorful fruits and vegetables, and complement them with lean proteins and whole grains.

Experiment with different cooking methods and flavors to keep your meals exciting and satisfying.

As you shop for groceries, remember that the perimeter of the store is often home to the freshest and most whole foods—produce, dairy, and lean meats. Venture into the aisles sparingly and with a discerning eye. Look for minimally processed options and whole-grain alternatives.

Eating Locally and Sustainably

Mindful eating transcends our individual well-being; it extends to the well-being of our planet and future generations. This is where the concept of eating locally and sustainably takes center stage. By making conscious choices about where our food comes from and how it is produced, we can reduce our environmental impact and support a more ethical and sustainable food system.

Eating locally involves sourcing your food from nearby farms and producers. When you choose local products, you not only support your local economy but also reduce the carbon footprint associated with transporting food over long distances. Additionally, local foods are often fresher and more flavorful, as they don't need to endure lengthy journeys to reach your plate.

Sustainable eating goes hand in hand with choosing foods that have been produced with the environment in mind. It means opting for products that have been grown or raised using practices that conserve natural resources, minimize pollution, and prioritize animal welfare. Sustainable choices can include organic produce, ethically raised meats, and seafood sourced from well-managed fisheries.

To practice mindful eating within a framework of sustainability, start by getting to know your local food scene. Visit farmers' markets, join community-supported agriculture (CSA) programs, and explore farm-to-table restaurants. Engage with local farmers and producers to learn about their practices and values. When dining out, seek out restaurants that prioritize locally sourced and sustainable ingredients.

Furthermore, consider reducing your meat consumption or exploring plant-based alternatives. The production of meat, particularly beef, has a significant environmental impact. By incorporating more plant-based meals into your diet, you can reduce your carbon footprint and support a more sustainable food system.

Building a mindful eating foundation through mindful food choices is about making informed, intentional decisions that align with your health, values, and the well-being of the planet. By understanding food labels, favoring whole and nutrient-dense foods, and embracing local and sustainable options, you not only nourish your body but also contribute to a more mindful and sustainable food culture. As you embark on this journey, remember that each choice you make brings you closer to a more vibrant and fulfilling relationship with food and the world around you.

3.3 Mindful Eating Environments

We've already explored the essence of understanding what mindful eating truly means and the physiological and psychological benefits it brings into our lives. As we continue to delve deeper into this transformative practice, we arrive at the pivotal aspect of creating the right environment to foster mindfulness during meals. Your surroundings play a significant role in how you experience food, and in this sub-chapter, we'll uncover the art of constructing a mindful eating environment—one that facilitates your connection with food and elevates your well-being.

Designing a Mindful Kitchen

Your kitchen isn't just a functional space; it's the heart of your mindful eating journey. It's where you prepare the ingredients that will nourish your body and soul. It's where you connect with the textures, aromas, and colors of your food. It's where you can either cultivate mindfulness or let it slip through your fingers.

Begin by decluttering your kitchen. Clear your countertops of unnecessary gadgets and appliances. A clutter-free space is a visual invitation to be present and focused. It allows you to breathe and move freely as you prepare your meals.

Consider the arrangement of your kitchen. Are your cooking utensils and ingredients easily accessible, or do you find yourself rummaging through cluttered drawers and cabinets? Arrange your kitchen so that everything you need for meal preparation is within arm's reach. This practical step minimizes distractions and allows you to stay in the moment.

Now, let's talk about lighting. Soft, warm lighting in the kitchen can create a cozy ambiance that encourages mindful eating. Harsh, fluorescent lighting can disrupt the sense of calm you're striving to create. Whenever possible, opt for natural light during the day, and in the evenings, use warm-toned bulbs to set the mood.

Plants can be your kitchen's best friends. They not only add a touch of nature but also purify the air, making the environment more pleasant and conducive to mindfulness. Keep a small herb garden on your windowsill, and you'll have fresh, aromatic herbs at your fingertips to elevate your culinary creations.

Mindful Dining Etiquette
As you progress on your mindful eating journey, the act of dining itself becomes an art form, a dance between you and your food. Mindful dining etiquette isn't about rigid rules; it's about embracing a set of practices that enhance your connection with your meals.

Begin with your seating arrangement. Choose a comfortable chair with good back support, ideally at a table that allows you to sit upright. Avoid dining on the couch or at your desk. Sitting at a table helps you maintain a posture that encourages mindful eating.

Set the table intentionally. Even if you're dining alone, place a cloth napkin neatly on your lap. Arrange your utensils, glass, and plate thoughtfully. These small actions create a sense of occasion and elevate your meal from a mere task to a sacred experience.

Put away your devices. In our modern world, it's tempting to scroll through social media or watch TV while eating. However, these distractions disconnect you from the present moment. Mindful eating is about engaging all your senses in the act of nourishing yourself. So, turn off the screens and be fully present with your food.

Chew your food thoroughly and savor each bite. Eating slowly not only allows you to taste the flavors more profoundly but also gives your body a chance to signal when you're full. It's a simple yet powerful practice that can prevent overeating.

Practice the art of conversation. If you're dining with others, engage in meaningful dialogue. Share your thoughts and experiences. Listening to others while you eat can help you slow down and appreciate your food more fully.

Eating with All Your Senses
Mindful eating is a multisensory experience, and to fully embrace it, you must engage all your senses. Each sense contributes to your understanding and enjoyment of food, making every meal a sensory adventure.

Start with sight. The presentation of your meal matters. Arrange your food on the plate with care, considering color, texture, and balance. A beautifully presented meal is not only visually appealing but also mentally satisfying.

Next, take in the aroma. Close your eyes and inhale deeply. Notice the subtle fragrances that waft up from your plate. Aromas play a vital role in your perception of flavor, so take the time to appreciate them before your first bite.

The sound of food can be surprisingly evocative. Listen to the sizzle of vegetables in a hot pan or the gentle bubbling of a simmering soup. Even the crunch of fresh produce can be a source of delight. These sounds can ground you in the present moment and amplify your connection to your meal.

Touch is a sense often overlooked in mindful eating, but it's no less important. Pay attention to the tactile qualities of your food. Feel the smooth skin of a ripe peach or the rough texture of whole-grain bread. Your fingertips are your first point of contact with your meal, so let them convey the story of your food.

And, of course, there's taste—the sense that takes center stage. As you take your first bite, close your eyes and savor the flavors. Let each taste bud on your tongue come alive. Notice the interplay of sweet, salty, sour, and bitter notes in your dish. Mindful eating is about tasting not just the food but the essence of each ingredient.

Incorporating all your senses into your eating experience transforms it from a mundane task into a sensory celebration. It deepens your appreciation for the food on your plate and reconnects you with the world around you.

The mindful eating environment you create has the power to transform your meals into moments of profound connection and nourishment. By designing a mindful kitchen, following mindful dining etiquette, and engaging all your senses, you pave the way for a more conscious and fulfilling relationship with food. It's not about perfection but about progress—a journey toward a more mindful, healthy, and joyful way of eating.

Chapter 4: Mindful Eating Practices

4.1 The Mindful Eating Ritual

Eating has become a rushed and often mindless activity in our hectic life. We hurriedly consume our meals while multitasking, barely pausing to taste the flavors or appreciate the nourishment our food provides. The result? We miss out on a profound opportunity for self-connection and well-being. But here's the good news: you can transform the way you eat by embracing the mindful eating ritual.

Setting the Stage for Mindful Meals

Imagine this: a beautifully set table, a carefully arranged plate of colorful and nutritious food, and the soothing ambiance of your favorite music playing softly in the background. This is the stage for a mindful meal, and it's far from ordinary.

The act of setting the stage for mindful meals is an essential component of the mindful eating ritual. It creates an atmosphere of intention and presence, signaling to your body and mind that this is a moment deserving of your full attention. Here's how you can do it:

1. Create a Sacred Space: Designate a specific area where you'll eat your meals. It could be your dining table, a cozy corner, or even a spot in your garden. Ensure it's free from distractions like television, phones, or work-related clutter.

2. Set the Table Mindfully: Lay out your tableware with care. Choose plates, utensils, and glasses that bring you joy and make you feel connected to the experience. Arrange them thoughtfully, perhaps with a simple centerpiece or a lit candle to add a touch of mindfulness.

3. Express Gratitude: Before you begin eating, take a moment to express gratitude. This can be a silent acknowledgment of the effort that went into preparing the meal, an appreciation for the food's origins, or simply a heartfelt "thank you" to yourself for taking this time to nourish your body.

By setting the stage for mindful meals, you are sending a powerful message to your subconscious that eating is not just a mundane task but a meaningful, even sacred, act of self-care and nourishment.

Savoring Every Bite

Have you ever finished a meal and realized you can barely recall what you just ate? You're not alone. Rushed eating often leaves us disconnected from the very experience of tasting and enjoying our food. But mindful eating invites you to savor every bite, making each meal a sensory delight.

Savoring is more than simply chewing your food slowly; it's about engaging all your senses to fully experience the flavors, textures, and aromas of your meal. Here's how you can savor every bite mindfully:

1. Engage Your Senses: As you take your first bite, close your eyes and focus on the flavors. Notice the sweetness, saltiness, or spiciness. Pay attention to the texture—Is it crunchy, creamy, or tender? Inhale deeply to capture the aroma of your food.

2. Chew Slowly and Thoughtfully: Put your fork or spoon down between bites. Chew each mouthful thoroughly, savoring the taste. Notice how the food transforms as you chew, releasing its full flavor.

3. Silence Your Inner Critic: Release any judgments or critical thoughts about your food. Instead, embrace an attitude of curiosity and non-judgment. Every meal is an opportunity to explore new tastes and textures.

4. Express Appreciation: Take moments during your meal to express appreciation for the nourishment and pleasure your food brings. You might silently say, "This is delicious," or "I am grateful for this meal."

5. Mindful Pauses: Pause between bites. Put your utensil down and take a breath. Check in with your body—Are you still hungry? Are you satisfied? This simple pause helps you listen to your body's cues.

By savoring every bite, you not only derive greater pleasure from your meals but also cultivate a deeper connection to your body's signals of hunger and satisfaction. This practice can help you avoid overeating and make more conscious choices about what and how much you eat.

Avoiding Distractions

We live in a world filled with distractions, and the dinner table is often no exception. The TV blares in the background, smartphones ping with notifications, and our minds wander to the stresses of the day. Mindful eating requires that we break free from these distractions and bring our full attention to the act of nourishing ourselves.

Avoiding distractions is a conscious choice, and it's one that can profoundly impact your relationship with food. Here's how you can do it:

1. Silence Your Devices: Commit to turning off or silencing your phone during meals. Use this time as an opportunity to disconnect from the digital world and reconnect with yourself.

2. Create a No-Screen Zone: Designate your dining area as a screen-free zone. This means no TV, no laptops, and no tablets at the table. Make it a rule for yourself and your family.

3. Practice Mindful Eating Silence: Invite silence into your meals. While it's natural to engage in conversation during dinner, consider dedicating the first few minutes to eating in silence. This allows you to fully focus on the sensory experience of your food.

4. Mindful Breathing: If your mind starts to wander during a meal, gently bring your attention back to your breath. Take a deep breath in and exhale slowly. This centers you in the present moment.

5. Mindful Conversations: If you do engage in conversation during meals, practice mindful listening. Give your full attention to the person speaking, and when you respond, do so with intention and presence.

Avoiding distractions during meals may initially feel challenging, but with practice, it becomes a powerful way to cultivate mindfulness. It allows you to fully appreciate the food in front of you and the company you're sharing it with.

Incorporating the mindful eating ritual into your daily life takes time and patience, but the rewards are immeasurable. By setting the stage for mindful meals, savoring every bite, and avoiding distractions, you'll not only transform your relationship with food but also embark on a journey of self-discovery and holistic well-being. Each meal becomes an opportunity to nourish not only your body but also your soul.

4.2 Mindful Portion Control

In the journey toward achieving your ideal body through mindful eating, one of the fundamental aspects to master is portion control. In our world of super-sized meals and calorie-packed snacks, it's easy to lose track of what constitutes a reasonable portion. However, by embracing the principles of mindful portion control, you can take charge of your eating habits and pave the way for effective weight management and a healthier relationship with food.

Understanding Portion Sizes

Before we delve into the mindfulness aspect of portion control, let's begin with a basic understanding of what portion sizes actually are. Have you ever found yourself looking at a plate of food and wondering, "Is this too much? Is it enough?" You're not alone. Portion sizes have grown significantly over the years, and what we see on our plates today is often far more than what our bodies actually need.

Portion control starts with awareness. It's about recognizing what a healthy portion looks like for different types of foods. For instance, a serving of lean protein like chicken or tofu should be about the size of your palm. A single serving of grains, like rice or pasta, should roughly equate to the size of your closed fist. And when it comes to vegetables, load up your plate generously; they're low in calories and packed with nutrients.

Now, here's where mindfulness comes into play. Instead of simply following strict measurements and rules, mindful portion control encourages you to engage your senses and intuition. When serving yourself, take a moment to look at your plate. Does it seem balanced? Does it appear excessive? By trusting your instincts and paying attention to visual cues, you can adjust your portions to align with your body's actual needs.

Mindful Eating and Weight Management

Mindful eating goes hand in hand with weight management. It's not about restrictive diets or depriving yourself of the foods you love; instead, it's a practice that fosters a healthy relationship with food and an understanding of your body's hunger and fullness signals.

When you practice mindful portion control, you're less likely to overeat. Mindful eaters savor each bite, paying attention to the flavors and textures of their food. This heightened awareness enables you to recognize when you're satisfied and when you've had enough, preventing that uncomfortable feeling of being overly full.

Consider this scenario: You're at a restaurant, and your meal arrives, piled high on the plate. A non-mindful eater might feel obligated to finish everything simply because it's there. But a mindful eater will take a few moments to assess their hunger and eat until they feel comfortably satisfied, regardless of the portion size. This approach not only prevents overeating but also supports gradual and sustainable weight management.

It's important to remember that weight management isn't solely about restriction; it's about making choices that align with your goals and honoring your body's signals. Mindful portion control empowers you to do just that. It encourages you to enjoy your food without guilt and make choices that contribute to your overall well-being.

Avoiding Overeating

The art of avoiding overeating is a crucial skill in mindful portion control. Overeating can feel like a thief in the night, robbing you of the satisfaction and comfort food should bring. It leaves you feeling bloated, guilty, and questioning your self-control. But there's a way to fortify yourself against this common pitfall: mindfulness.

Mindful eating requires you to slow down and truly experience your food. It's about being present in every moment, from the first bite to the last. When you engage in this level of awareness, it becomes challenging to overeat. You become acutely attuned to the sensations in your body, and as soon as your stomach signals that it's had enough, you're ready to put down your fork.

Here's a practical tip to avoid overeating: start with smaller portions. Instead of piling your plate high, serve yourself a moderate amount. You can always go back for seconds if you're still hungry. This simple act trains your mind to be mindful of your intake and to honor your body's cues.

Another powerful tool is eating slowly. Picture yourself at a leisurely dinner with a dear friend. You engage in conversation, enjoying each other's company, and savoring the meal in front of you. The pace is unhurried, allowing you to appreciate the flavors, textures, and aroma of each bite. This is the essence of mindful eating. By chewing slowly, you give your stomach time to communicate with your brain and let it know that it's time to stop eating when you're full.

Moreover, it's essential to recognize the emotional aspects of overeating. Sometimes, we turn to food as a coping mechanism for stress, boredom, or other emotions. Mindful eating encourages us to become detectives of our own behaviors. When you find yourself reaching for that second or third helping, pause and ask yourself if it's physical hunger or an emotional craving. By acknowledging your emotions and addressing them without food, you take a giant step towards avoiding overeating.

In the world of mindful eating, there's no judgment. There's only understanding and empowerment. So, if you slip up and overeat occasionally, that's okay. Mindful portion control isn't about perfection; it's about progress. It's about building a healthier relationship with food one mindful bite at a time. Remember, you have the power to choose the portion sizes that nourish your body and support your well-being.

4.3 The Mindful Eating Challenge

In the journey toward mastering mindful eating, we come across various challenges that test our commitment and discipline. These challenges often arise from our environment, emotions, and social situations. But fear not; with the right strategies and mindset, you can overcome them and continue reaping the benefits of mindful eating.

Mindful Eating in Social Situations

Social gatherings, family dinners, and outings with friends can be both delightful and daunting when you're committed to mindful eating. It's easy to get swept up in the excitement, lose track of what you're consuming, and abandon your mindful eating practices. So, how can you navigate these situations mindfully and enjoy them to the fullest?

Key Point 1: The Power of Conscious Choice

The first step in practicing mindful eating in social situations is to make a conscious choice about your approach. You can decide to fully indulge in the experience, savoring each bite and relishing the social aspect of sharing a meal with loved ones. Alternatively, you can choose to be more selective, opting for healthier options and smaller portions. The key is to make this choice deliberately and without guilt.

Key Point 2: Mindful Preparation

Before you step into the social scene, take a moment to mentally prepare. Visualize yourself practicing mindfulness during the event. Imagine yourself calmly choosing foods that nourish your body and savoring each bite without judgment. This mental rehearsal can help you stay aligned with your mindful eating goals.

Key Point 3: Set Clear Boundaries

Communicate your mindful eating goals with those you're sharing the meal with, if you feel comfortable doing so. Explain that you're making conscious choices about your food, not as a restriction but as an act of self-care. Setting these boundaries can lead to a more supportive and understanding environment.

Overcoming Cravings and Emotional Triggers
Cravings and emotional triggers are formidable opponents on the path of mindful eating. They often lead us to mindlessly reach for comfort foods when we're stressed, sad, or overwhelmed. But there's a way to break free from this cycle and regain control over your choices.

Key Point 1: Mindful Craving Awareness

The first step in overcoming cravings is to become fully aware of them. When a craving strikes, pause for a moment. Instead of immediately giving in, take a deep breath and ask yourself if you're truly hungry or if it's an emotional craving. Recognizing the nature of your craving is the first step to conquering it.

Key Point 2: Distract and Delay

Once you've identified a craving as emotional rather than physical hunger, employ distraction techniques. Engage in a brief mindfulness exercise, such as focused breathing or a short meditation. Alternatively, occupy your mind with an enjoyable non-food-related activity for a set period, say 15 minutes. Most often, the craving will dissipate during this time, and you'll regain control over your choices.

Key Point 3: Substitute Mindful Indulgences

Indulging in comfort foods doesn't have to be entirely off-limits. Instead, substitute unhealthy choices with mindful indulgences. If you're craving something sweet, opt for a piece of dark chocolate with a hint of sea salt. If it's a salty snack you desire, roasted almonds or air-popped popcorn can satisfy the craving in a healthier way.

Staying Consistent with Mindful Eating
Consistency is the cornerstone of any successful mindful eating practice. Yet, life's unpredictability can throw curveballs our way. Whether it's a hectic schedule, travel, or simply a busy day, staying consistent with mindful eating requires adaptability and resilience.

Key Point 1: Prioritize Planning

Planning is your best ally in staying consistent. Begin your day with a mindful breakfast, even if the rest of your day is uncertain. Pack healthy snacks and a balanced lunch if you'll be away from home. Having mindful options readily available reduces the chances of mindless choices when hunger strikes.

Key Point 2: Mindful Eating on the Go

Travel and dining out often challenge our commitment to mindful eating. In these situations, it's essential to maintain your awareness and make thoughtful choices. Explore local cuisine with mindfulness, choose whole-food options, and savor the experience without overindulging. Remember, you can still enjoy the flavors of a new culture while staying aligned with your mindful eating goals.

Consistency doesn't mean perfection. There will be times when you slip up or circumstances force you to deviate from your ideal mindful eating plan. In these moments, practice self-compassion. Acknowledge that setbacks happen to everyone and use them as opportunities for growth. The most important thing is to recommit to mindful eating as soon as possible and move forward with resilience.

The mindful eating journey is a path filled with challenges, but each challenge is an opportunity for growth and self-discovery. In social situations, cravings, and times of inconsistency, you can maintain your commitment to mindful eating through conscious choices, awareness, and self-compassion. By mastering these aspects of mindful eating, you'll find yourself better equipped to navigate life's complexities while nurturing a healthier and more harmonious relationship with food.

Chapter 5: Mindful Eating for Weight Management

5.1 Mindful Eating for Weight Loss

In our relentless pursuit of the "perfect" body, we often embark on weight loss journeys with grand expectations and fad diets. We chase the elusive mirage of rapid weight loss, only to find ourselves back where we started, or even further behind. It's time to shift our perspective and embrace a sustainable approach: mindful eating for weight loss.

Setting Realistic Weight Loss Goals

First and foremost, let's talk about setting realistic weight loss goals. The journey toward a healthier, happier you begins with clear intentions. We often want to shed pounds rapidly, envisioning ourselves in that dream dress or fitting into those old jeans. While it's admirable to have ambitions, it's crucial to temper them with realism.

Weight loss is not a one-size-fits-all equation. Your body is unique, and your weight loss journey will be too. Instead of aiming for a specific number on the scale, focus on achievable milestones. Set goals like "losing 1-2 pounds per week" or "increasing my daily steps." These targets are not only attainable but also sustainable.

Mindful eating encourages you to connect with your body's cues. As you embark on your weight loss journey, pay close attention to your hunger and fullness signals. Eat when you're hungry, stop when you're satisfied. It may sound simple, but it's a profound shift from mindless munching to conscious consumption.

Consider journaling your food intake, emotions, and physical sensations. This practice can help you identify triggers for overeating and provide valuable insights into your eating habits. Remember, the journey to weight loss is not solely about the destination; it's about understanding and nurturing your body along the way.

Mindful Eating as a Sustainable Weight Loss Strategy
Now, let's delve into why mindful eating is not just another diet but a sustainable weight loss strategy. Traditional diets often involve strict rules, deprivation, and unsustainable restrictions. They set us up for a cycle of losing and gaining, also known as "yo-yo dieting."

Mindful eating, on the other hand, fosters a healthy relationship with food. It's not about what you can't eat but about embracing a more mindful approach to what you can. It encourages you to savor each bite, to enjoy the flavors and textures of your meals, and to eat with intention.

When you approach your weight loss journey mindfully, you're more likely to make conscious food choices. You become attuned to your body's needs and are less likely to turn to emotional eating. Mindful eating empowers you to distinguish between physical hunger and emotional hunger, helping you break free from the cycle of using food as comfort.

Let's face it; diets are often unsustainable because they're built on restriction. But mindful eating allows room for indulgence. It's not about completely eliminating your favorite treats; it's about savoring them in moderation. When you enjoy that piece of chocolate or slice of pizza consciously, you're less likely to overindulge out of guilt or deprivation.

Another valuable aspect of mindful eating for weight loss is the ability to identify and address mindless eating patterns. These are those moments when you eat out of habit, without thinking. It's the bag of chips you finish while watching TV or the candy you mindlessly grab from your desk at work. By recognizing these patterns, you can develop strategies to interrupt them.

For instance, if evening snacking is a recurring habit, try this: Before reaching for a snack, take a few deep breaths and ask yourself if you're genuinely hungry. If the answer is yes, opt for a nutritious and satisfying option. If it's no, find an alternative activity to engage your mind or body.

Furthermore, mindful eating is a long-term commitment to your well-being. It's a lifestyle change, not a quick fix. It's about building a lasting foundation for healthier eating habits that will serve you well not just in your weight loss journey but throughout your life.

Here's a practical exercise: Before each meal, pause for a moment and assess your hunger on a scale from 1 to 10, with 1 being ravenous and 10 being uncomfortably full. Aim to start eating when you're around a 3 or 4 and stop when you reach a 6 or 7. This simple practice can work wonders for weight management by preventing overeating.

Adjust Mindful Eating Based on Your Achievement
As you embark on your mindful eating journey for weight loss, it's essential to remain flexible and adaptable. Remember that your needs and circumstances may change as you progress toward your goal.

As you make headway, you might discover that your hunger cues become more attuned, or that emotional eating no longer has the same grip on you. This is the perfect time to adjust your mindful eating practices. Perhaps you can gradually introduce more intuitive eating, where you trust your body's signals to guide your food choices.

Additionally, as you shed excess weight, you might want to focus on specific nutritional goals. For example, increasing your intake of fiber-rich foods like vegetables and whole grains can help you feel full and satisfied with fewer calories. Likewise, ensuring you consume an adequate amount of lean protein can support muscle retention as you lose weight.

However, it's vital to approach these adjustments with caution and continue to prioritize the principles of mindfulness. Avoid slipping into rigid dieting mentality or excessive restriction. Mindful eating encourages a balanced, intuitive approach to food, where no food is inherently "good" or "bad."

Furthermore, remember that weight loss isn't solely about the number on the scale. It's about overall health and well-being. As you progress on your mindful eating journey, celebrate your achievements along the way. Celebrate not only the pounds lost but also the improved relationship you've cultivated with food, the enhanced awareness of your body's signals, and the empowerment you've gained over your eating habits.

Mindful eating is a powerful and sustainable strategy for weight loss when approached with realistic goals, practiced consistently, and adapted to your evolving needs. It's about embracing a balanced and compassionate relationship with food, where you make choices that nourish both your body and your soul. So, embark on this journey with patience, self-compassion, and the knowledge that you have the capacity to transform your relationship with food and achieve your weight loss goals in a mindful and meaningful way.

5.2 Mindful Eating for Weight Maintenance

Welcome to the second part of our exploration into mindful eating for weight management. In the previous sub-chapter, we delved into the journey of mindful eating for weight loss. But as you may know, the real challenge lies not just in shedding those pounds but also in keeping them off. This sub-chapter is all about maintaining the ideal body you've worked so hard to achieve and preventing the dreaded weight regain. We'll also guide you through creating a mindful maintenance plan that sets you up for long-term success.

Maintaining Your Ideal Body

You've reached your weight loss goal, and it's an incredible achievement. But what comes next? Maintaining your ideal body weight is a journey in itself. The truth is, it's often more challenging than the initial weight loss. You've learned to navigate the world of mindful eating during your weight loss journey, and now, it's about making those practices a seamless part of your everyday life.

One of the key principles of mindful eating for weight maintenance is to remain consistent. Keep applying the mindfulness techniques that got you to your goal weight. Continue to eat slowly, savoring each bite, and paying attention to your body's signals of hunger and fullness. But remember, it's not about being overly restrictive. Allow yourself some flexibility and the occasional indulgence while keeping a keen eye on portion sizes.

Mindful maintenance is about finding your balance. It's recognizing that the journey is not over, but it's also not an endless cycle of dieting. This is where the transition from a weight loss mindset to a maintenance mindset is crucial. You're no longer solely focused on shedding pounds; you're now invested in a lifestyle that keeps you healthy and at your ideal weight.

It's essential to stay mindful of your triggers and potential pitfalls. Emotional eating, stress, and environmental influences can still affect your eating habits. By identifying these triggers and using the mindfulness techniques you've honed, you can continue to make conscious choices that support your ideal body.

Preventing Weight Regain

One of the most significant concerns after weight loss is the fear of regaining the lost pounds. It's a legitimate concern, but with mindfulness, you have a powerful tool to help prevent weight regain.

Mindful eating encourages you to stay connected to your body's signals. It's about listening to what your body needs, not what your cravings dictate. When you've reached your ideal weight, it's crucial to continue paying attention to hunger and fullness cues. Many people make the mistake of returning to old eating habits once they've lost weight, which inevitably leads to regaining those pounds.

To prevent weight regain, establish a support system. Share your goals and progress with friends or family who understand and respect your commitment to mindful eating. Having a support network can make a world of difference when faced with temptations or challenges.

Another strategy is to set clear boundaries. While you can indulge occasionally, it's essential to define what "occasionally" means to you. Create guidelines that help you stay on track without feeling overly restrictive. For example, you might decide that you'll enjoy dessert at social gatherings but won't keep sweets in your home to avoid mindless snacking.

Remember that regular physical activity is also a critical component of weight maintenance. Exercise helps you maintain muscle mass and keeps your metabolism in check. Mindfully incorporate physical activity into your routine, just as you've done with your eating habits. Find activities you enjoy to make it sustainable in the long term.

Creating a Mindful Maintenance Plan
Now, let's get practical about creating a mindful maintenance plan that will serve as your compass on this journey. Your plan should be personalized to fit your preferences, lifestyle, and needs. Here's how you can build one that works for you:

1. Set Realistic Goals: Your maintenance plan should begin with setting clear, realistic goals. Consider what maintaining your ideal body weight means to you. Is it about sustaining a certain number on the scale, feeling healthy and energized, or fitting into a specific clothing size? Define your objectives clearly.

2. Establish a Meal Routine: Continue to eat mindfully by sticking to a regular meal routine. Plan your meals and snacks to avoid unnecessary gaps in your eating schedule, which can lead to overeating later. Consistency is key.

3. Keep a Food Journal: Maintaining a food journal can help you stay accountable. Record what you eat, when you

eat, and how you felt before and after eating. This practice will help you identify any patterns or triggers that might lead to mindless eating.

4. Practice Mindful Grocery Shopping: Be selective about the foods you bring into your home. Shop mindfully, focusing on whole, nutrient-dense foods. When you have a well-stocked kitchen with healthy options, it becomes easier to make mindful choices.

5. Stay Active: Don't let physical activity fall by the wayside. Incorporate exercise into your daily routine, just as you did during your weight loss journey. Find activities you enjoy, whether it's dancing, hiking, or practicing yoga.

6. Monitor Your Progress: Regularly assess your progress and make adjustments as needed. If you notice your weight trending in the wrong direction, take it as an opportunity to reevaluate your mindful eating practices and activity level.

Mindful eating for weight maintenance is about sustaining the healthy habits you've developed while allowing room for flexibility and self-compassion. It's not about perfection but about creating a lifestyle that supports your ideal body. By staying mindful of your choices, triggers, and goals, you can enjoy the benefits of a healthier, happier, and more balanced life.

5.3 Mindful Eating and the Role of Mindset

In the realm of mindful eating, we often find ourselves navigating the complex terrain of our own thoughts and emotions. It's a journey where the connection between body and mind plays a pivotal role, especially when it comes to weight management. In this sub chapter, we're delving into the profound impact of mindset on weight management, exploring mindful body positivity practices, and shifting our focus from mere appearance to the overarching realm of health.

The Impact of Mindset on Weight Management

Let's begin by acknowledging a fundamental truth: our minds hold immense power. The way we perceive ourselves and our bodies can significantly influence our behaviors, including how we approach food and exercise. It's no secret that society often bombards us with images of what we're supposed to look like – svelte, toned, and seemingly flawless. The pressure to conform to these ideals can lead to a skewed perception of our own bodies.

Consider, for a moment, the impact of a negative mindset. When we constantly berate ourselves for not measuring up to societal standards, it becomes challenging to establish a healthy relationship with food. The guilt, shame, and self-doubt that often accompany negative self-talk can become barriers to mindful eating. We may find ourselves seeking solace in unhealthy eating habits or even resorting to extreme diets in a desperate attempt to meet these unrealistic ideals.

However, by shifting our mindset to one of self-compassion and self-acceptance, we can transform our relationship with food. Mindful eating encourages us to treat ourselves with kindness and understanding. It teaches us to let go of judgment and embrace the present moment. When we replace self-criticism with self-love, the choices we make concerning our diet and lifestyle become healthier, more balanced, and aligned with our overall well-being.

So, how can you cultivate a positive mindset in your mindful eating journey? It starts with recognizing and challenging negative thought patterns. When you catch yourself thinking unkind thoughts about your body or eating habits, take a moment to pause. Consider whether these thoughts are rooted in reality or influenced by external pressures. By becoming aware of these patterns, you gain the power to replace them with more constructive and compassionate thoughts.

Mindful Body Positivity Practices
Mindful eating is not just about what you consume; it's about how you perceive yourself in relation to your food and your body. Body positivity, a concept that has gained momentum in recent years, aligns beautifully with mindful eating. It's about accepting and appreciating your body, regardless of its shape or size.

Incorporating body positivity practices into your daily routine can have a profound impact on your relationship with food and, ultimately, your weight management journey. Start by fostering gratitude for your body. Consider all the remarkable things it enables you to do — from enjoying a walk in the park to embracing loved ones in a warm hug. By shifting your focus to what your body can do rather than what it looks like, you create a positive foundation for mindful eating.

Moreover, try to silence the inner critic. We all have that voice inside us, whispering doubts and insecurities. The key is not to eliminate it entirely (because let's face it, that's a tall order), but rather to become more adept at ignoring it when it chimes in. Acknowledge the negative self-talk, then consciously choose to redirect your thoughts toward self-compassion and acceptance.

Another invaluable body positivity practice is to surround yourself with positive influences. Engage with people, media, and communities that promote self-love and acceptance. By immersing yourself in a culture of body positivity, you reinforce these ideals in your own life. Remember, you are the sum of the influences you allow into your world, so curate it thoughtfully.

Shifting Focus from Appearance to Health
In the age of filtered selfies and airbrushed images, it's easy to get caught up in the pursuit of an idealized appearance. But here's a secret: the concept of an "ideal" body is highly subjective and often unattainable. It's a moving target that can leave you perpetually dissatisfied.

Mindful eating invites you to shift your focus away from appearance and toward health. Instead of obsessing over numbers on a scale or a clothing size, consider how you feel – both physically and mentally. Are you energized and alert? Do you feel confident and happy in your own skin? These are the markers of true health.

The truth is, health is not a one-size-fits-all concept. It varies from person to person and can't be distilled into a single set of measurements or standards. Therefore, striving for health should never be about conforming to someone else's idea of what's healthy. It's about understanding your own body's needs and nurturing them.

When you shift your focus to health, mindful eating becomes a means to an end – the end being a vibrant and fulfilling life. It's about nourishing your body with foods that make you feel strong and energetic, not depriving yourself to meet an arbitrary weight goal. This shift in perspective empowers you to make choices that support your long-term well-being.

But let's be clear: this doesn't mean abandoning the idea of managing your weight altogether. Rather, it means approaching weight management from a holistic perspective. When health is your primary focus, you're more likely to make sustainable, nourishing choices. It's not about restriction; it's about balance and self-care.

The mindset you bring to your mindful eating journey is a powerful determinant of your success. By cultivating a positive and compassionate mindset, embracing body positivity practices, and shifting your focus from appearance to health, you pave the way for a sustainable and fulfilling approach to weight management. Remember, it's not about perfection; it's about progress and self-acceptance. Your journey is uniquely yours, and the destination is a healthier, happier you.

Chapter 6: Mindful Eating for Emotional Well-being

6.1 The Emotional Eating Connection

Emotions are an intrinsic part of the human experience. They color our world, drive our actions, and, quite significantly, influence our eating habits. The complex interplay between emotions and eating is what this chapter aims to unravel. We'll delve into the emotional eating connection, helping you identify those triggers that lead you to the fridge, the ways in which mindful eating can become your armor against emotional turmoil, and how, ultimately, you can build emotional resilience that sets you free from the shackles of emotional eating.

Identifying Emotional Triggers

Emotional eating often begins with a trigger—a feeling, an event, a thought that sends you in search of comfort in the form of food. These triggers can vary greatly from person to person and can even change within an individual over time. They might be external, such as stress at work, a disagreement with a loved one, or even a celebratory event. Or, they can be internal, manifesting as loneliness, sadness, boredom, or anxiety.

Understanding Your Triggers

To tackle emotional eating, start by understanding your own triggers. Self-awareness is your greatest ally here. Keep a journal to track your eating patterns and jot down your feelings before and after each meal. This will help you uncover patterns and identify the specific emotions that lead to your unplanned trips to the kitchen.

The Mindful Self Question

Once you've identified your emotional triggers, the next step is to create a mindful self question before reaching for food. When you feel that familiar urge to eat in response to an emotion, take a moment to pause. Close your eyes, take a deep breath, and ask yourself: "Am I truly hungry, or am I seeking solace in food?" This simple act of pausing and questioning can be remarkably effective in breaking the automatic link between emotions and eating.

Using Mindful Eating to Manage Emotions

Mindful eating is a powerful tool in managing your emotions without turning to food for solace. It involves paying full attention to the present moment, the sensations of eating, and the emotions that arise during the process. Here's how you can use mindful eating to navigate the treacherous waters of emotional turmoil:

Embrace the Full Experience

When you sit down to eat, make it a ritual. Engage all your senses. Observe the colors and textures of your food, inhale its aroma, and savor each bite slowly. By immersing yourself fully in the eating experience, you divert your attention away from troubling emotions and toward the nourishment in front of you.

Learn to Recognize Physical vs. Emotional Hunger

Mindful eating helps you become attuned to your body's signals. You can differentiate between physical hunger and emotional hunger. Physical hunger builds gradually and is often felt in the stomach, while emotional hunger tends to strike suddenly and is usually accompanied by specific cravings. By recognizing these distinctions, you can respond appropriately. When it's emotional hunger, try engaging in a non-food-related activity to address the emotion instead.

Practice Mindful Coping Strategies

Mindful eating isn't just about how you eat; it extends to how you cope with emotions. Instead of reaching for food as your default coping mechanism, experiment with other mindfulness-based strategies. Meditation, deep breathing exercises, or even a brief walk can help you process emotions in a healthier way.

Building Emotional Resilience

Emotional resilience is the cornerstone of overcoming emotional eating. It's the ability to bounce back from adversity, to adapt to life's challenges without losing your sense of self. Here's how you can build emotional resilience on your mindful eating journey:

Cultivate Self-Compassion

The road to emotional resilience starts with self-compassion. Treat yourself with the same kindness and understanding that you would offer to a dear friend. Understand that emotions are a natural part of life, and it's okay to experience them. Avoid self-criticism for turning to food in the past; instead, focus on your commitment to change.

Seek Support and Connection

Building emotional resilience doesn't mean you have to do it all alone. In fact, seeking support and connection is a sign of strength. Share your struggles with trusted friends, family members, or a therapist who can provide guidance and a listening ear. Connecting with others who have faced similar challenges can also be incredibly empowering.

Practice Mindfulness Meditation

Mindfulness meditation isn't just a tool for managing emotions in the moment; it's a practice that can help you build emotional resilience over time. Regular meditation sessions can teach you to observe your thoughts and emotions without judgment, allowing you to respond to them more skillfully.

Set Realistic Goals and Expectations

Resilience isn't about never experiencing difficult emotions; it's about bouncing back when you do. Set realistic goals and expectations for yourself on your mindful eating journey. Understand that there will be setbacks, and that's perfectly normal. What matters is your commitment to keep moving forward, learning from your experiences, and growing stronger.

Learn from Your Emotional Eating Episodes

Each time you find yourself succumbing to emotional eating, view it as an opportunity for growth. Instead of berating yourself, reflect on what triggered the episode and how you could have responded differently. Use these moments as valuable lessons on your path to greater emotional resilience.

The emotional eating connection is a complex web of triggers, habits, and emotions. However, armed with mindfulness and emotional resilience, you have the power to break free from its grip. By identifying your emotional triggers, using mindful eating as a coping strategy, and building emotional resilience, you can transform your relationship with food and emotions, ultimately leading to greater well-being and a healthier, happier you.

6.2 Mindful Eating and Stress Reduction

Stress is an unwelcome companion that often sits at our dining table. It lurks in the corners of our minds, whispering to us, and sometimes screaming, to turn to comfort foods when life gets tough. It's the reason why you may find solace in that extra slice of cake or a bag of chips during moments of stress. But there's a way out of this cycle, and it involves a practice that goes beyond the plate and deep into the core of our emotions – mindful eating.

The Role of Stress in Overeating

Let's start by addressing the elephant in the room: stress-induced overeating. We've all been there, haven't we? A tough day at work, an argument with a loved one, or simply feeling overwhelmed can lead us to the kitchen in search of comfort. It's a phenomenon known as emotional eating, and it's a slippery slope.

When stress takes the reins, our brains often seek solace in high-calorie, high-sugar, and high-fat foods. Why? Well, it's because these foods trigger the release of feel-good neurotransmitters like dopamine. In the short term, they make us feel better. But in the long term, they can wreak havoc on our health and well-being.

Mindful eating steps in as the first line of defense against stress-induced overeating. It encourages us to pause, to acknowledge our emotions, and to consider alternative ways of coping with stress that don't involve raiding the cookie jar. By bringing awareness to our thoughts and feelings around food, we can make more conscious choices, even in moments of stress.

Imagine this scenario: You've had a tough day at work, and the only thing you can think about is that bag of chips in the pantry. Instead of diving right in, you pause. You take a few deep breaths and ask yourself, "Am I truly hungry, or am I seeking comfort?" This simple act of mindfulness can help you recognize the emotional trigger and choose a healthier way to deal with it, such as going for a walk or practicing a brief meditation.

Mindful Eating Techniques for Stress Relief

Now that we've acknowledged the role of stress in our eating habits, let's explore how mindful eating techniques can become your stress-relief arsenal. These techniques aren't just about what's on your plate; they're about transforming the entire eating experience into a mindful ritual.

1. Slow Down and Savor - In the midst of stress, our tendency is to rush through meals, barely tasting the food as it disappears from our plates. Mindful eating encourages us to slow down and savor each bite. Take the time to appreciate the textures, flavors, and aromas of your meal. Engage your senses fully. You'll find that this simple act of slowing down can be a calming balm for your frayed nerves.

2. Mindful Breathing - Stress often leads to shallow, rapid breathing. But you can use your breath as a tool to anchor yourself in the present moment. Before you start your meal, take a few moments to engage in mindful breathing. Inhale deeply through your nose, allowing your abdomen to expand, and then exhale slowly through your mouth. This conscious act of breathing can help lower stress levels and create a sense of calm.

3. Portion Control - Mindful eating isn't just about what you eat; it's also about how much you eat. Pay attention to portion sizes and avoid overloading your plate. When stress tempts you to overindulge, remind yourself that smaller, well-balanced portions can provide the same satisfaction without the guilt or discomfort of overeating.

4. Remove Distractions - We're all guilty of eating in front of the TV or computer, scrolling through our smartphones, or engaging in other distractions during meals. When it comes to mindful eating, it's time to unplug. Create a designated eating space free from distractions, and fully focus on your meal. You'll be amazed at how much more enjoyable and satisfying your food becomes.

5. The Power of Gratitude - Stress often makes us fixate on what's going wrong in our lives. Counteract this by practicing gratitude before each meal. Take a moment to reflect on the journey your food has taken to reach your plate – the farmers, the cooks, the harvesters. By acknowledging the effort that went into your meal, you can shift your focus from stress to appreciation.

Achieving Balance in Your Life
While mindful eating techniques can help manage stress in the moment, achieving a balanced and stress-resilient life requires a more holistic approach. Mindful eating is just one piece of the puzzle, albeit an essential one.

Consider this: Stress isn't solely caused by external factors; our internal reactions to those factors play a significant role. Mindfulness extends beyond the dining table and into every aspect of our lives. By cultivating mindfulness as a way of being, you can transform your relationship with stress.

1. Mindfulness Meditation - A regular mindfulness meditation practice can be a game-changer in stress

management. It's not about emptying your mind of thoughts but rather observing those thoughts without judgment. This practice enhances your ability to respond to stressors calmly and rationally instead of reacting impulsively.

2. Mindful Movement - Physical activity is an excellent stress reliever, but the key is to engage in it mindfully. Whether it's yoga, tai chi, or simply going for a walk, focus on the sensations in your body, your breath, and the present moment. This mindful approach to exercise can amplify its stress-reducing benefits.

3. Prioritize Self-Care - In the rush of daily life, self-care is often the first thing sacrificed. Yet, it's during stressful times that self-care becomes even more critical. Make time for activities you enjoy, be it reading, gardening, or simply taking a long bath. These moments of self-care can recharge your emotional batteries.

4. Seek Support - You don't have to navigate the complexities of stress alone. Share your feelings with a trusted friend, family member, or therapist. Talking about your stressors can provide perspective and emotional relief.

Achieving balance in your life is about integrating mindfulness into your daily routine. It's a journey that requires patience and practice, much like mindful eating itself. As you continue to explore the interplay between stress and mindful eating, remember that every meal is an opportunity to nourish your body and soul, to find solace in the present moment, and to cultivate resilience in the face of life's challenges.

6.3 Mindful Eating and Mental Health

In our fast-paced world, we often overlook the deep connection between what we eat and how we feel emotionally. The foods we consume can significantly impact our mental health, affecting our mood, energy levels, and overall well-being. It's a connection that's often underestimated but holds immense power to transform our emotional landscape. In this subchapter, we will explore the profound relationship between mindful eating and mental health, delving into how it can help alleviate anxiety and depression and offering holistic approaches to nurture our emotional well-being.

Mindful Eating and Anxiety

Anxiety, the silent but pervasive companion of many, can sometimes feel like an insurmountable mountain. Racing thoughts, a pounding heart, and a sense of impending doom can take over, leaving you feeling helpless. But what if I told you that the power to soothe your anxious mind might be right on your plate? It's time to explore the link between mindful eating and anxiety, and how the choices we make can either fuel or alleviate our worries.

When we're anxious, our body's stress response kicks into high gear. Cortisol, the stress hormone, floods our system, urging us into a fight-or-flight mode. It's in these moments that our food choices can either exacerbate or mitigate our anxiety. Mindful eating encourages us to pause and assess our emotions before diving into that bag of chips or pint of ice cream. By doing so, we become more aware of our triggers and our habitual responses to stress.

Consider this scenario: You've had a particularly stressful day at work, and all you want is comfort food. Instead of mindlessly indulging, try this mindful approach. Stop for a moment. Breathe. Acknowledge your anxiety. Now, choose a healthier option, such as a cup of herbal tea or a small serving of dark chocolate. By making a conscious choice, you regain a sense of control over your emotions and your food.

Moreover, the types of foods we consume can play a pivotal role in managing anxiety. Foods rich in omega-3 fatty acids, like salmon and flaxseeds, have been linked to reduced anxiety symptoms. Antioxidant-rich fruits and vegetables, such as blueberries and spinach, can help combat oxidative stress and inflammation associated with anxiety. These choices not only nourish your body but also your mind, providing essential nutrients to keep anxiety at bay.

Mindful eating also encourages us to savor our meals slowly, appreciating the flavors and textures. This practice can be particularly beneficial for anxiety, as it redirects your focus away from racing thoughts and towards the present moment. It's a simple yet powerful technique to help you stay grounded and centered during challenging times.

As you navigate your mindful eating journey, remember
that it's not about perfection but progress. Small changes in
your food choices and eating habits can lead to significant
improvements in anxiety management. Each mindful bite is
a step towards a calmer, more balanced emotional state.

Mindful Eating and Depression

Depression, like a heavy cloud, can cast a shadow over our
lives, making even the simplest tasks seem insurmountable.
While mindful eating may not be a magical cure for
depression, it can be a valuable tool in your arsenal to
alleviate some of its symptoms and support your mental
well-being.

When depression takes hold, it often leads to changes in
appetite and eating patterns. Some may turn to food for
comfort, resulting in overeating or consuming unhealthy,
processed foods. Others may experience a loss of appetite,
leading to inadequate nutrition and energy levels. Mindful
eating seeks to restore a healthier relationship with food,
one that nourishes both the body and the mind.

One of the key principles of mindful eating is self-
compassion, something that individuals grappling with
depression often lack. Depression can be incredibly
isolating, and self-criticism can become a relentless
companion. Mindful eating gently encourages you to treat
yourself with kindness and understanding, to recognize that
your struggles do not define your worth.

Imagine this: You wake up in the morning, and the weight of depression feels particularly heavy. The thought of breakfast may seem daunting, but you decide to practice mindfulness. You prepare a simple, nourishing meal—a bowl of oatmeal with fresh fruit. You sit down at the table, focusing on the warmth of the bowl in your hands and the aroma of the food. You take one bite at a time, savoring each spoonful. In this moment, food becomes a source of solace and self-care rather than a source of guilt or shame.

Moreover, the nutrients we obtain from food play a vital role in brain health and can influence mood and cognition. Foods rich in vitamins, minerals, and antioxidants, such as leafy greens, nuts, and whole grains, provide essential support to the brain. They can help regulate neurotransmitters like serotonin and dopamine, which are closely linked to mood and motivation.

Holistic Approaches to Mental Health
While mindful eating offers valuable strategies to address anxiety and depression, it's essential to acknowledge that mental health is a multifaceted journey. Holistic approaches encompass a range of practices and principles that can complement mindful eating, creating a comprehensive plan for emotional well-being.

1. Meditation and Mindfulness: Regular meditation practice can enhance your capacity to manage stress and reduce symptoms of anxiety and depression. Mindfulness meditation, in particular, aligns beautifully with the

principles of mindful eating, as it cultivates awareness and presence in all aspects of life.

2. Exercise: Physical activity is a natural mood lifter. It releases endorphins, your brain's feel-good neurotransmitters, which can help combat symptoms of depression. Incorporating mindful exercise, like yoga or tai chi, adds an extra layer of emotional support.

3. Sleep Hygiene: Prioritizing quality sleep is crucial for mental health. Establishing a sleep routine and creating a relaxing bedtime ritual can contribute to more restful sleep, which in turn, can alleviate symptoms of depression and anxiety.

4. Social Connection: Human connection is a fundamental aspect of well-being. Engaging in meaningful social interactions and seeking support from loved ones or a therapist can be an essential part of your holistic approach to mental health.

5. Professional Help: When depression and anxiety become overwhelming, seeking professional guidance is a brave and vital step. Mental health professionals can provide therapy, medication, or a combination of both to support your journey towards emotional well-being.

In the realm of mindful eating and mental health, we embark on a journey of self-compassion and self-care. The choices we make at the table can empower us to navigate the complex terrain of anxiety and depression. As we practice mindful eating, we discover the profound connection between nourishing our bodies and nurturing our minds. You have the power to transform your relationship with food and, in doing so, transform your emotional landscape. With mindful eating as your ally, you can find the strength and resilience to embrace a life rich in well.

Chapter 7: Mindful Eating for Special Diets

7.1 Mindful Eating for Vegetarians and Vegans

In a world where dietary choices abound, the decision to embrace a vegetarian or vegan lifestyle is a profound one. It's a choice driven by compassion for animals, a concern for the environment, and a pursuit of better health. But with these choices come the responsibilities of meeting your nutritional needs mindfully, exploring the diverse world of plant-based cuisine, and mastering the art of mindful meal planning for plant-based diets.

Meeting Nutritional Needs Mindfully

Transitioning to a vegetarian or vegan diet is not just about eliminating animal products; it's also about ensuring that you receive all the necessary nutrients to thrive. It's common for people to worry about protein intake when they make this switch, but rest assured, a well-balanced plant-based diet can provide ample protein. The key is to approach this transition mindfully.

One of the primary concerns is getting enough protein. Plants offer a variety of protein sources, from legumes like lentils, chickpeas, and beans to tofu, tempeh, and seitan. Nuts and seeds, such as almonds, chia seeds, and hemp seeds, are also protein-packed. Be mindful of including a variety of these sources in your diet to ensure you get a wide spectrum of amino acids.

Iron is another nutrient that often raises concerns. While plant-based iron (non-heme iron) isn't as easily absorbed as iron from animal sources (heme iron), you can enhance absorption by consuming iron-rich foods alongside vitamin C sources. For instance, pair your iron-fortified cereals with a glass of orange juice or add strawberries to your morning oatmeal.

Calcium is essential for strong bones, and many people associate it primarily with dairy products. However, there are plenty of plant-based sources of calcium, such as fortified plant milks (like almond, soy, or rice milk), tofu, leafy greens (kale and collard greens), and sesame seeds. Mindfully incorporating these into your diet ensures you meet your calcium needs.

Vitamin B12 is a nutrient that deserves special attention for vegans, as it's primarily found in animal products. To meet your B12 requirements, consider fortified foods like plant milks, breakfast cereals, and nutritional yeast. Some vegans also choose to take B12 supplements to ensure they're getting enough.

Omega-3 fatty acids, important for heart and brain health, can be sourced from flaxseeds, chia seeds, walnuts, and hemp seeds. However, consider algae-based supplements for a more reliable source of EPA and DHA, which are typically found in fish.

In the realm of mindful eating, being aware of your nutrient intake and making informed choices is paramount. Regularly monitor your nutrient levels through blood tests to ensure you're meeting your needs, and don't hesitate to consult with a registered dietitian who specializes in plant-based nutrition to tailor your diet to your unique requirements.

Exploring Plant-Based Cuisine

One of the most exciting aspects of adopting a vegetarian or vegan lifestyle is the opportunity to explore a world of diverse and delicious plant-based cuisines. You'll find that there's a wealth of flavors, textures, and cultural influences to savor. Embrace this journey with an open heart and an adventurous palate.

Mediterranean cuisine, with its abundance of fresh vegetables, olive oil, and herbs, provides a rich tapestry of flavors. Explore dishes like tabbouleh, hummus, and falafel. These dishes are not only incredibly tasty but also packed with nutrients.

Indian cuisine offers a wide array of vegetarian and vegan options. Dive into flavorful curries made with lentils, chickpeas, or tofu. Savor the aromatic spices that define Indian cooking, such as cumin, coriander, and turmeric.

Thai cuisine is another gem for plant-based eaters. Dishes like vegetable green curry, pad Thai with tofu, and spicy coconut soups will tantalize your taste buds.

Japanese cuisine is known for its simplicity and balance. Enjoy vegetable sushi rolls, miso soup, and tempura vegetables. The umami-rich flavors of seaweed, soy sauce, and miso paste take center stage.

Mexican cuisine offers a plethora of vegetarian and vegan options. Savor dishes like bean burritos, vegetable fajitas, and guacamole. Explore the tangy and spicy flavors that Mexican cuisine is famous for.

Mediterranean, Indian, Thai, Japanese, and Mexican cuisines are just the tip of the iceberg. The world is your culinary playground, and as a mindful eater, you have the privilege of savoring diverse and nutritious plant-based dishes from every corner of the globe.

Mindful Meal Planning for Plant-Based Diets
Meal planning is a cornerstone of mindful eating, and it becomes even more critical when you adopt a vegetarian or vegan diet. Planning ahead ensures that you have balanced meals that provide the nutrients your body needs to thrive.

Start by setting aside time each week for meal planning. Take a look at your schedule and decide which meals you'll cook at home and which you'll eat out or order in. Having a plan reduces the chances of resorting to convenience foods that may not align with your dietary goals.

When planning your meals, aim for variety. Incorporate different grains like quinoa, brown rice, farro, and whole wheat pasta. Mix up your protein sources, rotating between beans, lentils, tofu, tempeh, and plant-based meat substitutes if you choose.

Plan your meals around vegetables. Aim to fill at least half your plate with colorful, nutrient-rich vegetables. Think about the rainbow of colors you can include – red tomatoes, orange carrots, green broccoli, purple eggplant, and more.

Experiment with recipes from different cuisines to keep your meals exciting. Try making a weekly menu that includes Italian, Mexican, Thai, and Mediterranean-inspired dishes.

Consider batch cooking and meal prep. Spending a few hours on the weekend preparing ingredients or entire meals can save you time and make it easier to stick to your plant-based eating plan during busy weekdays.

Don't forget to include healthy snacks in your meal plan, such as fresh fruit, nuts, or veggie sticks with hummus. These can help curb hunger between meals and prevent less mindful snacking on less nutritious options.

Lastly, listen to your body. Mindful eating is not just about what you eat but also about how your body responds to it. Pay attention to hunger and fullness cues, and adjust your portion sizes accordingly.

As you venture into the world of plant-based eating, remember that mindful eating is a powerful ally on your journey. By meeting your nutritional needs mindfully, exploring diverse plant-based cuisines, and crafting thoughtful meal plans, you can thrive on a vegetarian or vegan diet. Embrace this new way of nourishing yourself with open-mindedness, curiosity, and a love for all the flavors the plant kingdom has to offer.

7.2 Mindful Eating for Allergies and Intolerances

In our diverse world, dietary restrictions are not uncommon. Food allergies and intolerances affect millions of people, making mealtime a minefield of potential hazards. But here's the good news: with the right approach, it's possible to navigate this terrain mindfully, ensuring your health and well-being while still enjoying delicious, safe, and satisfying meals. In this sub-chapter, we'll delve deep into the art of mindful eating for those with food allergies and intolerances.

Navigating Food Allergies Mindfully

First and foremost, let's talk about food allergies. Living with a food allergy can feel like walking on eggshells, but with mindfulness as your guide, you can confidently navigate the culinary world. The key is awareness.

Begin by becoming a label detective. When you're at the grocery store, don't rush through the aisles. Take your time to read ingredient labels meticulously. Look for common allergens like peanuts, tree nuts, dairy, soy, and wheat. The food industry has come a long way in terms of allergen labeling, so you'll often find clear warnings if a product contains any of these allergens.

However, remember that labels can be deceiving. Cross-contamination is a real concern in food processing facilities. If a product isn't labeled as allergen-free but doesn't contain the allergen in its ingredient list, proceed with caution. Many brands now offer dedicated allergen-free product lines, making your job easier.

Eating out at restaurants can be a minefield. But being mindful doesn't mean you have to avoid dining out altogether. When choosing a restaurant, do your research in advance. Many restaurants now publish allergen menus online. Call ahead and speak to the staff about your dietary needs. A restaurant that takes your allergies seriously will appreciate your proactive approach and ensure a safe dining experience.

Practice assertive communication. When you're ordering, clearly and calmly communicate your allergies to your server. Don't be shy about asking questions or requesting modifications to dishes. It's your health, after all. Mindful eating means advocating for yourself and your well-being.

Mindful Shopping for Allergy-Friendly Foods
Shopping mindfully for allergy-friendly foods isn't just about scrutinizing labels; it's also about embracing the world of whole, unprocessed foods. When you're dealing with food allergies, the fewer ingredients in a product, the better. Natural, unprocessed foods are your allies.

Fresh produce is your safe haven. Fruits, vegetables, and herbs are naturally allergen-free. Embrace the rainbow of flavors and textures they offer. When selecting grains, opt for gluten-free alternatives like quinoa, rice, or oats specifically labeled as gluten-free to avoid cross-contamination.

Don't forget about the treasure trove of legumes. Lentils, chickpeas, and beans can be the foundation of satisfying, allergen-friendly meals. Nuts and seeds are often fine for those with nut allergies; just be sure to source them from a reputable supplier with clear allergen information.

Dairy allergies or lactose intolerance? Explore the world of plant-based milks, such as almond, soy, or oat milk. These alternatives have come a long way in terms of taste and texture, making them excellent dairy substitutes in both cooking and baking.

When it comes to cooking oils and condiments, stick with the basics. Olive oil, coconut oil, and avocado oil are typically safe bets. For condiments, check labels carefully or consider making your own. Homemade sauces and dressings not only give you full control over ingredients but also taste better than their store-bought counterparts.

Cooking and Dining Safely
Now, let's dive into the heart of mindful eating for those with food allergies or intolerances: the kitchen. Cooking mindfully is your ultimate safeguard against accidental exposures. It's not just about what you cook but how you cook it.

Create an allergy-free zone in your kitchen. This designated space ensures that allergen-containing foods and utensils never cross-contaminate your safe cooking area. Consider color-coding cutting boards, utensils, and cookware to minimize the risk further.

When preparing meals, follow this golden rule: clean, clean, clean. Wash your hands, utensils, and cooking surfaces thoroughly before you begin. Cross-contamination can occur easily if you're not diligent.

Mindful cooking also means selecting recipes that align with your dietary needs. Thankfully, countless resources are available today for allergen-friendly cooking. Explore cookbooks, blogs, and cooking apps dedicated to your specific allergies or intolerances. You'll discover a world of flavorful recipes designed with you in mind.

And remember, cooking allergen-friendly doesn't mean sacrificing taste. Experiment with herbs, spices, and alternative ingredients to create dishes bursting with flavor. The world of culinary creativity is at your fingertips.

When it's time to dine, approach your meal with a sense of calm and mindfulness. Before taking the first bite, pause and take a moment to express gratitude for the safe and nourishing food in front of you. Savor each mouthful, paying attention to the textures and flavors. This moment of mindfulness not only enhances your dining experience but also helps you detect any potential issues promptly.

In social settings, such as potlucks or gatherings, don't hesitate to bring your own dish to ensure you have a safe option. Share your dietary needs with your host, and if you're dining out, contact the restaurant in advance to discuss your allergies or intolerances.

Navigating food allergies and intolerances mindfully is not just a necessity; it's an empowering journey. By practicing awareness, assertive communication, and mindful cooking and dining, you reclaim control over your culinary experience. Remember, your dietary restrictions don't define your enjoyment of food; they enhance it. Approach each meal with gratitude, mindfulness, and the knowledge that you can savor every bite while safeguarding your health.

7.3 Mindful Eating for Special Health Conditions

When it comes to mindful eating, one of its most profound aspects is its adaptability. It's not a one-size-fits-all approach but rather a versatile tool that can be harnessed to address specific health conditions. In this sub-chapter, we will delve into how mindful eating can be a transformative ally for individuals managing diabetes, aiming for heart health, and nurturing digestive wellness.

Mindful Eating for Diabetes Management

Diabetes, a condition that affects millions worldwide, requires vigilant management of blood sugar levels. But what if I told you that mindfulness could be a game-changer in this journey? The truth is, it can. Mindful eating brings a heightened awareness to your eating habits, allowing you to make choices that promote stable blood sugar levels and overall well-being.

Key Point 1: Understanding Your Body

Mindful eating begins with understanding your body's unique responses to different foods. When you have diabetes, your body's ability to regulate blood sugar is compromised. This means that certain foods can cause rapid spikes in blood sugar levels, while others may have a gentler effect. To harness the power of mindful eating, start by keeping a food journal. Record what you eat and monitor how your body responds. Over time, patterns will emerge, helping you identify which foods are your allies and which are your adversaries.

Key Point 2: The Mindful Art of Portion Control

One of the primary challenges for individuals with diabetes is managing portion sizes. Mindful eating equips you with a potent tool to conquer this challenge. Before you dive into a meal, pause and take a moment to appreciate the food in front of you. Assess your hunger cues. Are you eating because it's mealtime, or are you genuinely hungry? Once you start eating, savor each bite, chew slowly, and put your fork down between bites. This allows your body to send signals of fullness to your brain, preventing overeating and helping to control blood sugar levels.

Key Point 3: Choosing Mindfully, Every Time

Mindful eating for diabetes is not a temporary diet but a lifelong commitment to making mindful choices. It means selecting foods that are low on the glycemic index—foods that release glucose into the bloodstream gradually. These include whole grains, vegetables, lean proteins, and legumes. When you shop, read food labels attentively, and be on the lookout for hidden sugars and carbohydrates. Remember, mindfulness is not about deprivation but about making choices that serve your long-term health.

Mindful Eating and Heart Health

Our hearts are the engines that keep us going, and maintaining heart health is a fundamental aspect of overall well-being. Enter mindful eating, a practice that can significantly impact heart health by promoting balanced eating habits and encouraging choices that benefit your cardiovascular system.

Key Point 1: Savor the Good Fats

One of the keys to heart health is consuming healthy fats while avoiding the unhealthy ones. Mindful eating encourages you to savor foods rich in heart-healthy fats, such as avocados, nuts, and olive oil. These fats have been shown to reduce the risk of heart disease when consumed in moderation. However, portion control is crucial here too, as fats are calorie-dense. Pay attention to your body's signals to avoid overindulging.

Key Point 2: Mindful Sodium Intake

Excessive sodium intake can lead to high blood pressure, a significant risk factor for heart disease. Mindful eating helps you keep your sodium consumption in check by making you more conscious of the foods you choose. When you're mindful of your choices, you're less likely to opt for processed foods high in sodium. Instead, you'll gravitate toward whole, unprocessed foods that are naturally lower in sodium and healthier for your heart.

Key Point 3: Balancing Macros for Heart Health

The balance of macronutrients in your diet plays a pivotal role in heart health. Mindful eating prompts you to think about your meals in terms of balance. Your plate should ideally include a lean source of protein, a variety of colorful vegetables, and whole grains. This combination provides a wide range of nutrients that support heart health. Additionally, fiber-rich foods like beans and oats help lower cholesterol levels, reducing the risk of heart disease.

Mindful Eating and Digestive Health
Your digestive system is not just responsible for processing the foods you eat; it plays a critical role in overall health. Digestive issues can lead to discomfort and negatively impact your quality of life. Fortunately, mindful eating can help you cultivate better digestive health.

Key Point 1: Slow Down for Optimal Digestion

Digestion begins in your mouth, where enzymes in your saliva start breaking down food. When you eat too quickly, you bypass this essential initial step. Mindful eating encourages you to savor each bite, chew thoroughly, and eat at a relaxed pace. This simple practice can alleviate digestive discomfort and enhance nutrient absorption.

Key Point 2: Choose Foods That Love Your Gut

A healthy gut is essential for good digestion. Certain foods, known as prebiotics and probiotics, can promote gut health. Prebiotics, found in foods like garlic, onions, and asparagus, provide nourishment for beneficial gut bacteria. Probiotics, found in fermented foods like yogurt and kimchi, introduce these friendly bacteria into your digestive system. Mindful eating guides you to incorporate these gut-loving foods into your diet, supporting a happy, healthy digestive system.

Key Point 3: Listen to Your Body's Signals

Your body has an intricate system of signals that tell you when to eat and when to stop. Mindful eating encourages you to tune in to these signals. When you eat mindfully, you're more likely to eat when you're hungry and stop when you're satisfied, rather than consuming excess food that your body doesn't need. This helps prevent overeating and reduces the risk of digestive discomfort.

Incorporating mindful eating into your life, whether you're managing diabetes, aiming for heart health, or nurturing digestive wellness, empowers you to take charge of your health with every bite. It's a practice that's not about rigid rules or restrictions but about creating a harmonious relationship between you and your food, leading to a healthier, happier you.

Chapter 8: Mindful Eating for Families

8.1 Teaching Children Mindful Eating

In the bustling cacophony of modern life, teaching children the art of mindful eating is like offering them a timeless gift—a gift that not only nurtures their bodies but also cultivates a deeper connection to the world around them. As a parent or caregiver, you hold the key to shaping your children's relationship with food, and in turn, their overall well-being. In this subchapter, we will delve into the essential practices of raising mindful eaters, establishing family mealtime rituals, and creating a nourishing food environment that fosters a lifelong appreciation for healthy eating.

Raising Mindful Eaters

Teaching children mindful eating begins with building a foundation of awareness, curiosity, and gratitude. It's about helping them recognize the beauty of each bite and the profound impact it has on their growing bodies. Here are some practical steps to guide you in raising mindful eaters:

1. Model Mindful Eating: Children are keen observers, and they often emulate the behaviors they see. Demonstrate mindful eating by savoring your meals, paying attention to the colors, textures, and flavors on your plate. Make it a point to eat together as a family whenever possible.

2. Encourage Exploration: Introduce a variety of foods to expand their palate and encourage them to explore different tastes and textures. Visit local farmers' markets or involve

them in meal preparation to pique their curiosity about the origins of food.

3. Teach the Five Senses: Help your children engage their five senses when eating. Encourage them to describe the taste, smell, texture, and appearance of the food. This sensory awareness enhances their appreciation for the culinary experience.

4. Practice Gratitude: Instill the practice of gratitude by expressing thanks for the food on the table. Share stories about the journey of food from farm to plate, fostering an appreciation for the effort that goes into providing nourishment.

5. Mindful Portions: Teach them about portion control without instilling a sense of restriction. Allow them to recognize their hunger and fullness cues. Encourage them to take second helpings if they're still hungry.

6. Avoid Food as a Reward or Punishment: Avoid using food as a reward for good behavior or withholding it as punishment. This helps prevent emotional connections to eating.

Family Mealtime Rituals
Family mealtime rituals are the cornerstone of mindful eating in a household. They provide a sense of togetherness, create a nurturing environment, and offer opportunities for meaningful conversations. Here are some ways to establish and cherish these rituals:

1. Set a Regular Schedule: Aim to have family meals at consistent times, whether it's breakfast, lunch, or dinner. Predictability offers comfort and structure to children.

2. Create a Welcoming Atmosphere: Set the stage for meals by dimming the lights, playing soothing music, or lighting candles. Make the dining area inviting and free from distractions like phones or TVs.

3. Practice Mindful Silence: Begin meals with a moment of silence or gratitude. Encourage each family member to reflect on the day and express appreciation for the food and each other.

4. Engage in Conversation: Use mealtime as an opportunity to engage in meaningful conversation. Encourage everyone to share their thoughts, experiences, and feelings. This practice promotes open communication and connection.

5. Family Cooking Time: Involve children in meal preparation. Let them participate in age-appropriate tasks, from washing vegetables to setting the table. It instills a sense of pride in contributing to the family's nourishment.

6. No Screens at the Table: Create a screen-free zone during meals. This rule fosters presence, allowing everyone to fully engage with the food and each other.

7. Mindful Chewing: Encourage slow and deliberate chewing. Discuss the importance of thoroughly enjoying each bite and digesting food properly.

Fostering a Healthy Food Environment
The environment in which children grow up profoundly influences their eating habits and choices. Creating a healthy food environment doesn't mean banishing all treats; instead, it's about striking a balance and offering a variety of nourishing options. Here's how you can foster such an environment:

1. Stock Nutrient-Dense Foods: Keep the pantry and fridge stocked with wholesome, nutrient-dense foods. When these options are readily available, children are more likely to choose them for snacks and meals.

2. Limit Processed Foods: Minimize the presence of heavily processed and sugary snacks in the house. Opt for whole fruits, vegetables, nuts, and seeds as go-to snacks.

3. Homemade vs. Store-Bought: Whenever possible, prepare meals and snacks at home. This not only allows you to control ingredients but also promotes the value of home-cooked meals.

4. Family Shopping Trips: Involve children in grocery shopping. Teach them to read food labels and make informed choices. Explain the importance of selecting fresh produce and whole grains.

5. Moderation is Key: While it's essential to offer a balanced diet, occasional treats are part of a healthy relationship with food. Teach children about moderation and enjoying indulgent foods mindfully.

6. Cook Together: Cooking together can be a bonding experience. Experiment with new recipes and ingredients as a family, encouraging a sense of culinary adventure.

7. Gardening Connection: If possible, consider planting a small garden together. Children gain a deeper appreciation for food when they witness its growth from seed to table.

8. Educational Approach: Explain the nutritional benefits of different foods without making it feel like a lecture. Engage children's curiosity by discussing how food fuels their bodies and minds.

9. Hydration Awareness: Encourage drinking water throughout the day and discuss the importance of staying hydrated for overall health.

Teaching children mindful eating is not a one-time endeavor but a lifelong journey. As they grow and mature, their understanding of food and their bodies will evolve. By imparting these valuable lessons and fostering a positive food environment, you're providing them with the tools to make informed, health-conscious choices in the years to come. Your influence as a parent or caregiver extends far beyond the dinner table, shaping their relationship with food and nourishment for a lifetime.

8.2 Mindful Eating for Busy Parents

Parenting is a magnificent journey, but it can also be an incredibly demanding one. Between diaper changes, school runs, work obligations, and countless other responsibilities, it's easy for parents to put their own well-being on the back burner. Yet, as any seasoned parent will tell you, maintaining your own health is not a luxury; it's a necessity. This sub chapter delves into the challenges busy parents face when trying to practice mindful eating and offers practical strategies for finding balance, nourishing your family, and taking care of yourself.

Balancing Work, Family, and Health

Balancing the demands of a career and a family can feel like walking a tightrope while juggling flaming torches. With schedules bursting at the seams, parents often resort to convenience foods or skip meals altogether. However, mindful eating is not just a hippie-dippie concept reserved for serene yoga instructors. It's a lifeline for busy parents.

Practical Tip 1: Meal Planning

One of the most effective ways to balance your work, family, and health is through meal planning. Sit down with your partner or family members and carve out some time each week to plan your meals. Take into account everyone's schedules, dietary preferences, and nutritional needs. When you have a plan, you're less likely to resort to unhealthy takeout or fast food on hectic nights.

Practical Tip 2: Bulk Cooking and Freezing

Sundays can be your meal prep day. Cook large batches of nutritious meals and freeze them in portions. On those nights when you're too tired to cook, you'll have a healthy option ready to go. It's like a home-cooked TV dinner, but without the mystery ingredients.

Practical Tip 3: Snack Smartly

Healthy snacking can be a busy parent's secret weapon. Stock up on easy-to-grab snacks like cut-up vegetables, fruit, yogurt, or nuts. These are not only convenient but also provide the nutrients your body needs to keep up with the whirlwind of parenthood.

Remember, mindful eating isn't about perfection; it's about intention. Even in the midst of chaos, you can choose to be mindful about what you and your family consume.

Quick and Healthy Meal Ideas
Time is often the scarcest resource for busy parents. Between school drop-offs, soccer practice, and work meetings, there never seems to be enough of it. But let's bust a myth right now: Healthy eating doesn't have to be time-consuming or complicated.

Practical Tip 1: Stir-Fry Suppers

Stir-fries are a busy parent's best friend. They're lightning-fast to make and offer endless variations. Grab some tofu, chicken, or tempeh, throw in a rainbow of veggies, and whip up a simple sauce with soy sauce, garlic, and ginger. Serve it over brown rice or quinoa, and voilà—an impressive, nutritious meal in under 30 minutes.

Practical Tip 2: One-Pot Wonders

Invest in a good-quality, large pot or slow cooker. With these kitchen heroes, you can create hearty soups, stews, and curries that simmer away while you go about your day. Load them up with vegetables, beans, or lentils for a balanced meal that practically cooks itself.

Practical Tip 3: Breakfast for Dinner

Break the traditional meal mold. Breakfast foods like scrambled eggs, whole-grain pancakes, or oatmeal with fresh berries and nuts can make for quick, wholesome dinners. Plus, kids usually love breakfast for dinner—it's a win-win.

When it comes to preparing healthy meals, efficiency is key. Keep it simple, focus on fresh ingredients, and let go of the idea that every meal has to be a culinary masterpiece. The goal is to nourish your family and yourself, not to become a Michelin-star chef.

Self-Care for Parents

As a parent, it's easy to get caught up in the whirlwind of taking care of everyone else and forget to care for yourself. However, self-care is not a luxury; it's a vital component of mindful eating and overall well-being.

Practical Tip 1: Prioritize Sleep

Sleep is the ultimate form of self-care for parents. It's when your body repairs, regenerates, and recharges. Set a bedtime routine for yourself just like you would for your kids. Create a sleep-conducive environment, turn off screens, and prioritize those precious hours of rest.

Practical Tip 2: Practice Mindful Snacking

In the chaos of parenthood, you might find yourself mindlessly munching on your child's leftover mac 'n' cheese or snacking on whatever's within arm's reach. Instead, take a moment to choose your snacks mindfully. Opt for something nutritious, and sit down to savor it. This moment of self-indulgence can be a mini-mindfulness meditation in itself.

Practical Tip 3: Delegate and Seek Support

You don't have to do it all alone. Don't hesitate to ask for help when needed. Whether it's sharing cooking duties with your partner or calling in reinforcements from grandparents or friends, accepting support is an act of self-care.

Practical Tip 4: Find Moments of Stillness

Mindful eating extends beyond the dining table. Find small moments of stillness throughout your day. Whether it's a few minutes of deep breathing, a short walk in the fresh air, or a moment of quiet contemplation, these pauses can help you stay grounded amidst the chaos.

Remember that you're not just a parent; you're a role model. By prioritizing self-care and mindful eating, you're not only nourishing yourself but also teaching your children valuable life skills. Parenthood is a marathon, not a sprint, and taking care of yourself is essential for the long haul.

8.3 Mindful Eating for Seniors

As we journey through life, our nutritional needs change, and nowhere is this transition more evident than in our senior years. The aging process is a natural part of life, but it comes with its unique challenges, including changes in metabolism, muscle mass, bone density, and overall health. However, mindful eating can be a powerful ally in ensuring that our golden years are filled with vitality and well-being.

Nourishing the Aging Body

Aging is a complex process, and our bodies evolve in numerous ways. Metabolism tends to slow down, which means we burn fewer calories. Muscle mass decreases, making it crucial to maintain strength through nutrition and exercise. Bone density also declines, increasing the risk of fractures. Hormonal changes may affect appetite and digestion. Chronic conditions become more prevalent.

Mindful eating offers a way to navigate these changes with grace and vitality. It starts with awareness. Being mindful of our changing bodies and unique nutritional requirements is the first step. It's about understanding that what nourished us in our younger years may no longer serve us as effectively. Instead of resisting these changes, we embrace them and adapt our eating habits accordingly.

Balanced Nutrition for Seniors

A balanced diet becomes even more critical in our senior years. This means prioritizing nutrient-dense foods that provide essential vitamins and minerals. It's about consuming a variety of colorful fruits and vegetables to ensure an array of antioxidants. Lean protein sources help maintain muscle mass, and healthy fats support brain health.

Mindful eating encourages us to savor each bite, appreciating the nourishment it provides. Slow, deliberate chewing aids digestion, which can be a concern for seniors. It allows us to listen to our bodies, to recognize when we're truly hungry and when we're satisfied, preventing overeating.

Hydration Matters

Staying adequately hydrated is vital, but it's easy for seniors to forget to drink enough water. Mindful eating encourages sipping water throughout the day, not just during meals. Infusing water with citrus or herbs can make it more appealing. Staying hydrated helps maintain cognitive function, digestive health, and overall well-being.

Addressing Age-Related Eating Challenges
The aging process can bring a host of eating challenges, some of which may require special attention. Mindful eating equips us with the tools to address these challenges head-on.

Chewing and Digestive Issues

Many seniors experience dental issues that can make chewing difficult. Others may face digestive problems, such as acid reflux or constipation. Mindful eating encourages us to choose foods that are easier to chew and digest. It emphasizes smaller, more frequent meals, reducing the burden on the digestive system.

Medications and Their Effects

Seniors often take medications for various health conditions. Some medications can affect appetite or taste perception. Mindful eating involves discussing these effects with healthcare providers and finding ways to adapt the diet accordingly. It may involve experimenting with new flavors or textures to make meals more appealing.

Social Isolation and Loneliness

Loneliness and social isolation can lead to changes in eating habits. Some seniors may lose interest in cooking or eating due to a lack of companionship. Mindful eating encourages social engagement around meals, whether through shared cooking or dining with friends and family. It reminds us that mealtime can be a source of connection and enjoyment.

Maintaining Independence Through Mindful Eating
One of the greatest concerns for seniors is maintaining their independence and quality of life. Mindful eating plays a vital role in ensuring that seniors can continue to enjoy autonomy in their food choices.

Meal Preparation and Planning

Cooking can become challenging as we age, but it doesn't have to be a burden. Mindful eating involves simplifying meal preparation while still prioritizing nutrition. It may mean using pre-cut vegetables, cooking in batches to have leftovers, or exploring meal delivery services. The focus is on finding convenient solutions that align with individual preferences.

Empowering Food Choices

Mindful eating empowers seniors to make choices that resonate with their tastes and values. It encourages them to explore new foods, try different cuisines, and savor the pleasures of eating. It reminds us that food is not just sustenance; it's a source of joy and nourishment.

Listening to the Body

Perhaps most importantly, mindful eating encourages seniors to listen to their bodies. It reminds them that hunger and fullness cues are reliable guides. Eating when hungry and stopping when satisfied is a simple yet powerful practice that supports independence and well-being.

In our senior years, the journey of mindful eating takes on a unique and profound significance. It becomes a path to embracing the changes that come with aging, nourishing our bodies, and maintaining the independence and vitality we cherish. As seniors, we recognize that mindful eating is not a rigid set of rules but a flexible and adaptive approach to nutrition. It allows us to savor the flavors of each meal, to appreciate the vibrant colors on our plates, and to nourish not just our bodies but also our spirits.

Through mindful eating, we navigate the challenges of aging with grace, resilience, and a deep sense of empowerment. We savor the simple pleasures of a well-prepared meal and the warmth of connection around the dinner table.

And as we continue this journey, we realize that mindful eating is not just a way to nourish our bodies—it's a path to nourishing our souls and savoring the richness of life in every bite.

Chapter 9: Mindful Eating and Culinary Creativity

9.1 The Art of Mindful Cooking

In the world of mindful eating, the kitchen is a sacred space—a canvas where we paint with flavors, textures, and colors to nourish not just our bodies, but our souls. The art of mindful cooking is about far more than preparing sustenance; it's an act of love, a form of self-expression, and a bridge that connects generations. In this sub chapter, we'll dive into the heart of mindful cooking, exploring how it can enhance the well-being and harmony of your family.

Embracing Culinary Creativity with Mindfulness

Picture this: a kitchen filled with the melodious sizzle of fresh ingredients hitting a hot pan, the aroma of garlic and herbs permeating the air, and the anticipation of a mouthwatering meal that will soon grace the table. This is the magic of culinary creativity, and when it's infused with mindfulness, it becomes an art form.

Mindful cooking begins with a profound appreciation for the ingredients you're working with. It's about touching, smelling, and truly seeing each component. As you chop, slice, and dice, you engage all your senses. The crispness of a bell pepper, the earthy scent of mushrooms, the vibrant hues of vegetables—all these sensations awaken you to the present moment.

When cooking becomes a mindful practice, it's no longer a hurried chore but a joyful ritual. It's about selecting ingredients mindfully, understanding their origins, and appreciating the effort that goes into cultivating them. As you immerse yourself in the process, you're more likely to make choices that align with your family's health and values.

Experimenting with Mindful Ingredients and Flavors
Mindful cooking is also about embracing experimentation. The culinary world is a treasure trove of ingredients and flavors waiting to be discovered. So, why not take your family on a flavor-filled adventure?

Consider the tantalizing world of spices. Cumin, paprika, turmeric, and cinnamon—they're more than just pantry staples; they're the keys to unlocking a world of taste sensations. By incorporating a variety of herbs and spices into your dishes, you not only add depth and character to your meals but also introduce your family to diverse cultures and culinary traditions.

When you explore new ingredients and flavors, you teach your children a valuable lesson: the world is vast, and there's beauty in its diversity. It's an opportunity to engage your family in conversations about different cuisines, traditions, and the importance of respecting and appreciating cultures beyond your own.

Don't be afraid to step outside your culinary comfort zone. Try your hand at creating dishes from various cuisines— Thai, Mexican, Indian, or Italian. Experiment with plant-based proteins like tofu, tempeh, or seitan. Introduce your family to the delights of vegetarian sushi rolls or the savory richness of a Mediterranean eggplant dish.

The essence of mindful cooking lies in approaching these culinary explorations with an open heart and an open mind. Allow your family to participate in selecting new ingredients or recipes to try. Turn it into a fun family activity, where everyone has a say in what's on the menu. Through these culinary adventures, you're fostering a sense of curiosity and a spirit of adventure in your children.

Mindful Cooking as a Form of Self-Expression
In our fast-paced lives, we often rush through meal preparation, treating it as a chore to be completed as quickly as possible. But what if we shift our perspective and see cooking as an opportunity for self-expression? Each dish you create can be a reflection of your love, creativity, and care for your family.

The act of mindful cooking allows you to infuse your energy into every bite. When you approach the stove with a sense of mindfulness, your state of mind and heart is transferred into the food you prepare. Your intention matters, and it's felt by those you cook for.

Mindful cooking can also be a form of self-care. It's a moment of solitude in a world that often demands constant attention. As you chop vegetables, stir sauces, and plate your creations, you're in the zone—a place where stress melts away, and time seems to stand still. This meditative aspect of cooking can be your daily retreat, a time to recharge and reconnect with yourself.

Involve your family in this journey of self-expression through food. Encourage your children to participate in age-appropriate tasks in the kitchen. Even the youngest members can help wash vegetables, arrange ingredients, or set the table. As they grow, involve them in more complex tasks, teaching them valuable life skills while strengthening the family bond.

Incorporate your family's preferences into the meals you create. If your child loves a particular vegetable, find creative ways to include it in your dishes. If someone prefers a certain cuisine, make it a family project to recreate those flavors at home. By doing so, you're not only expressing your love but also nurturing a sense of belonging and togetherness.

Mindful cooking is a celebration of the present moment, a canvas for culinary creativity, and a channel for self-expression. By infusing mindfulness into your family's cooking routine, you're not just nourishing their bodies; you're nourishing their souls and building lasting memories.

Embrace the beauty of mindful cooking as a family, and watch how it transforms your relationship with food, with each other, and with the world around you. It's a journey worth embarking upon, one that can enrich your family's lives in ways you never imagined. So, open your heart, sharpen your knives, and let the mindful cooking adventure begin.

9.2 Mindful Eating and Food Culture Exploration

In our quest to embrace mindful eating, there's a fascinating dimension that often goes unexplored: the world of culinary traditions and the rich tapestry of global flavors that await our senses. The journey toward mindful eating isn't merely about nourishing our bodies; it's about nurturing our souls through the diverse and delicious cuisines that cultures around the world have to offer. So, let's embark on a flavorful exploration of mindful eating and food culture, expanding our palates and our understanding of the world.

Exploring Global Culinary Traditions Mindfully

Have you ever wondered how people in different corners of the world approach food and meals? It's a profound journey of discovery that can broaden our horizons and deepen our connection to food. Mindful eating in the context of global culinary traditions involves not only savoring the flavors but also appreciating the cultural and historical significance behind each dish.

Take, for example, the Japanese tradition of kaiseki, a multi-course meal that celebrates seasonality, artistry, and the beauty of simplicity. Each meticulously prepared dish tells a story, inviting you to slow down, savor every bite, and engage your senses fully. When we approach kaiseki mindfully, we immerse ourselves in the culinary craftsmanship and the centuries-old rituals that have shaped this tradition.

Or consider the Mediterranean diet, celebrated for its health benefits and delectable flavors. It's a cuisine deeply rooted in the cultural practices of countries like Greece, Italy, and Spain. Mindful eating within this tradition means savoring the aroma of olive oil, the burst of freshness in a Greek salad, and the satisfaction of sharing a meal with loved ones under the Mediterranean sun. It's not just about the food; it's about the lifestyle and the communal spirit that accompanies it.

As you explore these culinary traditions and many others, you'll find that mindful eating transcends the boundaries of language. It becomes a universal language of appreciation, a way to connect with people from diverse backgrounds, and a means of forging bonds through the shared joy of food.

Mindful Dining as a Cultural Experience
Dining can be much more than the act of consuming calories; it can be a cultural experience that transports us to faraway lands and different time periods. When we embrace mindful dining within the context of cultural traditions, we not only nourish our bodies but also feed our curiosity and enrich our souls.

Imagine stepping into a traditional Indian restaurant, where the aroma of spices and the vibrant colors of curries and naan bread captivate your senses. Mindful dining here involves exploring the complex interplay of sweet, savory, and spicy flavors, all while acknowledging the rich history and spiritual significance of Indian cuisine. It's an opportunity to connect with the philosophy of balance and harmony that underlies Ayurveda and yoga, both deeply rooted in Indian culture.

Or perhaps you find yourself in a Moroccan riad, savoring the intricate flavors of a tagine—a slow-cooked stew infused with aromatic spices like cumin, cinnamon, and saffron. Mindful dining in Morocco means recognizing the art of hospitality and the importance of communal meals that bring families and friends together. It's about cherishing the rituals of sharing food, tea, and conversation in the company of loved ones.

Even if you can't travel to these far-flung places, you can bring the essence of these cultural experiences to your own dining table. Experiment with recipes, explore local international restaurants, or simply engage in conversations with people from diverse backgrounds. Every meal becomes an opportunity to embark on a culinary journey and deepen your appreciation for the cultural tapestry of our world.

Expanding Your Palate Mindfully

In the realm of mindful eating, expanding your palate is akin to embarking on an adventure—a thrilling voyage of taste, texture, and aroma. It's about challenging your taste buds and stepping out of your culinary comfort zone, all while remaining fully present in the moment.

One of the beautiful aspects of mindful eating is that it encourages us to be open to new experiences. It invites us to experiment with ingredients, spices, and dishes we may have never considered before. It's about giving your palate the gift of novelty and surprise.

Start by exploring your local international markets. Wander through the aisles and discover ingredients you've never seen or tasted. Pick up a spice you can't pronounce or a fruit you've never tried. The act of selecting these items mindfully, feeling their textures, and inhaling their scents, becomes an adventure in itself.

Next, take your newfound ingredients and embark on a culinary experiment. Try your hand at cooking a dish from a different culture. Whether it's preparing sushi rolls, whipping up a Thai curry, or making Spanish paella, the act of mindful cooking can be a meditation in itself. Pay attention to the colors, the sounds, and the transformation of raw ingredients into a flavorful masterpiece.

As you sit down to enjoy your creation, do so with full awareness. Take that first bite and let the flavors dance on your tongue. Notice the nuances and the way your taste buds respond to the new and exciting combination of tastes. This is the essence of expanding your palate mindfully— it's an exploration that keeps your culinary journey ever- evolving.

Incorporating mindful eating into the exploration of global culinary traditions not only enriches your gastronomic experiences but also fosters a deep sense of connection with the world. It's a reminder that, through food, we can bridge cultural gaps, celebrate diversity, and savor the beauty of our shared humanity.

So, embrace the world on your plate. Let each meal be an opportunity to travel, learn, and celebrate the kaleidoscope of flavors and cultures that our planet has to offer. Through mindful eating, you're not just nourishing your body; you're nourishing your soul, one delicious bite at a time.

9.3 Sharing Mindful Meals with Loved Ones

In a world often bustling with activity and noise, the act of sharing a mindful meal with loved ones can be a profound and transformative experience. It's a chance to connect on a deeper level, fostering relationships, and creating lasting memories. In this sub-chapter, we'll delve into the art of mindful eating in social gatherings, how to create meaningful connections through food, and the joy of hosting mindful dining experiences.

Mindful Eating in Social Gatherings

Imagine being at a vibrant gathering with friends and family. Laughter fills the air, and the aroma of delicious food wafts through the room. These occasions are not only about nourishing our bodies but also our souls. Mindful eating in social settings allows us to fully engage in the experience.

Key Point 1: Presence and Engagement

The first step to mindful eating in social gatherings is to be present. Put away distractions like your phone, take a deep breath, and fully engage with the people and food around you. When you're fully present, you're better able to savor the moment, the flavors, and the company.

Key Point 2: Savoring Each Bite

As you take that first bite, pay close attention to the flavors, textures, and aromas of the food. Let your taste buds dance to the tune of each dish. By savoring each bite, you not only enjoy the meal more but also become more attuned to your body's hunger and fullness cues.

Key Point 3: Mindful Conversations

Engaging in mindful conversations while eating can deepen your connections with others. Instead of discussing the latest news or your busy schedule, try sharing meaningful stories or expressing gratitude. Mindful conversations foster a sense of togetherness and create lasting bonds.

Creating Meaningful Connections through Food

Food has the incredible power to bring people together, transcending boundaries and cultures. It's a universal language that allows us to express love, celebrate life, and create shared memories. Here's how you can harness the potential of food to foster meaningful connections:

Key Point 1: Thoughtful Cooking and Gifting

Prepare meals for your loved ones with thought and care. Consider their preferences and dietary restrictions. Whether it's a homemade dinner or a batch of freshly baked cookies, the effort you put into creating a dish will be appreciated and remembered.

Key Point 2: Celebrating Traditions

Many cultures have unique food traditions tied to celebrations and gatherings. Embrace these traditions and share them with your loved ones. Whether it's a Japanese tea ceremony or an Italian pasta-making night, celebrating traditions through food adds depth to your connections.

Key Point 3: Food as an Expression of Love

Think about the times when someone prepared a meal just for you. It felt like an expression of love, didn't it? You can do the same for others. Cook with love, and let your food convey your affection and appreciation.

Hosting Mindful Dining Experiences

Hosting a mindful dining experience can be a wonderful way to share your love for food and mindfulness with others. It's an opportunity to create a space where people can connect, savor delicious dishes, and be present in the moment.

Key Point 1: Setting the Ambiance

Creating a mindful dining atmosphere is essential. Dim the lights, play soothing music, and set a beautifully arranged table. The ambiance you create sets the stage for a memorable experience.

Key Point 2: Mindful Menu Planning

When planning your menu, consider the flavors, textures, and colors of the dishes. Aim for a balanced meal that appeals to the senses. Incorporate fresh, seasonal ingredients to enhance the dining experience.

Key Point 3: Guided Mindfulness

During the meal, guide your guests through a mindfulness practice. Encourage them to take a moment of silence to appreciate the food before them. Lead them in a mindful breathing exercise to center themselves and fully engage in the meal.

Key Point 4: Encouraging Conversation

Promote meaningful conversations by providing conversation starters or discussion topics related to the meal. Encourage guests to share their thoughts on the flavors, ingredients, and memories associated with the dishes.

Key Point 5: Gratitude and Reflection

At the end of the meal, take a moment to express gratitude for the food, the company, and the moment shared. Encourage your guests to reflect on their experience and how mindful eating can be integrated into their daily lives.

Incorporating mindful eating into your social gatherings and culinary experiences can deepen your connections with loved ones and create a profound sense of togetherness. It's about more than just nourishing the body; it's about nourishing the soul. Embrace the opportunity to share mindful meals with others, and you'll find that the act of eating can become a powerful means of fostering meaningful connections.

Chapter 10: Integrating Mindful Eating with Exercise

10.1 The Mindful Exercise Connection

In the pursuit of a healthier, more vibrant life, the connection between mindful eating and exercise is the most important foundation. It's a dynamic synergy that, when understood and harnessed, can transform not just your body but your entire well-being. In this sub-chapter, we will delve deep into the Mind-Body Connection in Physical Activity, explore the concept of Mindful Movement, and uncover the incredible Benefits of Combining Mindful Eating and Exercise.

Understanding the Mind-Body Connection in Physical Activity

Exercise is often viewed as a means to an end, a path to achieving specific fitness goals, but it's so much more than that. It's a conversation between your mind and body, an exchange of energy and awareness that extends far beyond the confines of a gym or a yoga mat.

Think about the last time you engaged in a physical activity. Maybe it was a brisk walk, a yoga session, or even an intense weightlifting routine. Recall how your body responded as you moved, how your muscles engaged, your heart rate quickened, and your breath synchronized with your movements. These physical sensations are the language through which your body communicates with you.

Now, let's add mindfulness to the mix. When you approach exercise with mindfulness, you're not just going through the motions. You're fully present in your body, listening to its cues, and responding with care. This awareness elevates your exercise routine from a mundane task to a profound experience.

Imagine yourself practicing yoga, each pose a meditation in motion. As you transition from one asana to the next, you notice the subtle shifts in your balance, the stretch in your muscles, and the rhythm of your breath. Your mind is attuned to your body's signals, ensuring you don't push too hard or hold back unnecessarily.

In a mindful run, you feel the ground beneath your feet with every step, your senses alive to the world around you. The wind against your skin, the rhythm of your heartbeat, and the gentle ache in your muscles are all part of this conversation. You're not merely running; you're communing with your body and the environment.

This Mind-Body Connection is where the magic happens. It's where you learn to honor your body's limits, prevent injury, and find joy in movement. When you exercise mindfully, you're not fighting against your body; you're collaborating with it, nurturing it, and letting it guide you toward greater health.

Mindful Movement: A Holistic Approach to Exercise
We've all heard the phrase "No pain, no gain." It's a common mantra in the fitness world, often pushing people

to push harder, faster, and without regard for their bodies' signals. But what if we reframed this idea? What if we embraced the concept of "Know your body, achieve your goals"?

Mindful movement is about understanding that your body is a magnificent instrument, not a machine to be pushed to its limits. It's about acknowledging that exercise is not punishment but a celebration of what your body can do. It's a holistic approach that combines the wisdom of the mind with the physicality of the body.

In mindful movement, you set aside the notion of "working off" that last meal or "burning calories" as if they were debts to be repaid. Instead, you engage in physical activity as a way to nurture and care for your body. You move because it feels good, because it energizes you, and because it's an expression of self-love.

Consider a mindful walk in nature. As you step onto the trail, your intention is not to obliterate calories but to connect with the world around you. You listen to the birdsong, you feel the earth beneath your feet, and you breathe in the fresh air. This is exercise as a form of communion, a way to recalibrate your body and soul.

Mindful movement also means letting go of competition, whether with others or yourself. It's not about being the fastest, the strongest, or the most flexible person in the room. It's about being the best version of yourself, respecting your unique abilities, and embracing the journey.

When you approach exercise with this holistic mindset, you create a sustainable and enjoyable routine. It becomes something you look forward to, not a chore to check off your list. And as you cultivate this relationship with movement, you'll find that consistency and progress come naturally.

Benefits of Combining Mindful Eating and Exercise
Now that we've explored the Mind-Body Connection in Physical Activity and the concept of Mindful Movement, let's delve into the incredible Benefits of Combining Mindful Eating and Exercise. When you bring these two practices together, the synergy is nothing short of transformative.

1. Enhanced Physical Performance: Mindful eating provides your body with the nourishment it needs to excel in physical activities. By tuning in to your body's hunger and fullness cues, you optimize your energy levels, ensuring you're adequately fueled for your workouts. Imagine having the stamina to push through that extra set of reps or that final lap with ease.

2. Improved Recovery: After a strenuous exercise session, your body craves replenishment. Mindful eating helps you make wise choices in your post-workout meals, supplying your muscles with the nutrients they need to repair and grow. Your recovery time shortens, and you bounce back stronger than ever.

3. Weight Management: Combining mindful eating with exercise is a powerful tool for weight management. When you're aware of what you eat and why you eat, you're less likely to engage in emotional or mindless eating patterns. This means better control over your weight and a more balanced approach to fitness.

4. Reduced Stress: Both mindful eating and exercise have stress-reducing benefits. Mindfulness techniques can lower cortisol levels (the stress hormone), and exercise releases endorphins, those feel-good chemicals. Together, they create a potent antidote to the stresses of daily life.

5. Enhanced Mind-Body Connection: The Mind-Body Connection in Physical Activity is strengthened when combined with mindful eating. You become attuned to how different foods make you feel, allowing you to make choices that optimize your performance and overall well-being. Your exercise sessions become more intuitive, and you can fine-tune your routines based on how your body responds.

6. Long-Term Lifestyle Changes: Integrating mindful eating and exercise is not a quick fix; it's a sustainable lifestyle change. When you approach both practices with mindfulness, you build habits that endure. This isn't about temporary diets or workout fads; it's about embracing a way of life that promotes health and happiness.

Combining mindful eating with exercise is a holistic approach to well-being. It's not about perfection but about progress. It's about cultivating a relationship with your body that is rooted in self-compassion and self-care. And as you embark on this journey, you'll discover that the benefits extend far beyond your physical health; they permeate every aspect of your life, creating a balanced and ideal body and life.

10.2 Mindful Pre-Workout Nutrition

In the quest for a healthier, more balanced life, integrating mindful eating with exercise is a game-changer. It's not just about what you eat; it's about when and how you nourish your body. This subchapter delves into the first aspect of this synergy: mindful pre-workout nutrition.

Fueling Your Body Mindfully Before Exercise

Before you lace up your running shoes or step onto the yoga mat, it's essential to consider what your body needs for optimal performance. Mindful pre-workout nutrition isn't just about eating something; it's about making choices that will sustain your energy levels, boost endurance, and help you get the most out of your workout.

Key Point 1: The Right Balance of Macros

Mindful pre-workout nutrition begins with the right balance of macronutrients: carbohydrates, proteins, and fats. Carbohydrates are your body's primary source of energy, making them a crucial component of your pre-workout meal or snack. Opt for complex carbs like whole grains, sweet potatoes, or quinoa. These provide a slow and steady release of energy, preventing those mid-workout energy crashes.

Proteins play a role in muscle repair and growth, making them essential, too. A small amount of lean protein, such as tofu, tempeh, or Greek yogurt, can help prevent muscle breakdown during exercise.

Fats should be consumed in moderation before a workout. They take longer to digest, so opt for sources like avocado, nuts, or a drizzle of olive oil. These provide sustained energy without weighing you down.

Key Point 2: Portion Control

While it's important to fuel your body adequately, avoid overeating before exercise. A large meal can lead to discomfort during your workout. Instead, aim for a balanced, moderate-sized pre-workout snack or meal. Listen to your body and eat until you feel satisfied but not stuffed.

Key Point 3: Timing Matters

Timing your pre-workout meal or snack is crucial. Ideally, aim to eat about 1 to 3 hours before exercise. This gives your body enough time to digest and convert food into energy. If you're short on time, opt for a light, easily digestible snack, like a banana or a handful of almonds, about 30 minutes before your workout.

Optimal Pre-Workout Meal Timing and Choices
The concept of pre-workout nutrition isn't one-size-fits-all; it depends on the type, intensity, and duration of your exercise. Let's break down some scenarios and optimal choices for each:

1. Cardio Workouts: Running, Cycling, or Aerobics

For longer cardio workouts, aim for a balance of carbohydrates and a small amount of protein. A bowl of oatmeal with fresh berries or a whole-grain sandwich with lean protein and veggies can provide the right fuel. Ensure you eat at least an hour before your workout to allow for digestion.

2. Strength Training: Weightlifting or Bodyweight Exercises

Strength training benefits from a bit more protein in your pre-workout meal. Consider a veggie and tofu stir-fry with brown rice or a smoothie with protein powder, banana, and spinach. Eat about 2 hours before hitting the weights.

3. Yoga, Pilates, or Low-Intensity Workouts

For gentler workouts, keep your pre-workout nutrition light. A small piece of fruit or a handful of mixed nuts is sufficient to provide a little energy boost. Consume this snack about 30 minutes before your session.

Hydration and Exercise Performance

Nutrition isn't the only aspect of mindful pre-workout preparation; hydration plays a critical role, too. Proper hydration ensures that your body can perform at its best and helps prevent fatigue, cramps, and overheating.

Key Point 1: The Importance of Hydration

Starting your workout in a dehydrated state can hinder your performance and increase the risk of injury. It's essential to begin your exercise session well-hydrated. In the hours leading up to your workout, aim to sip water regularly. The goal is to maintain a pale, straw-colored urine, indicating proper hydration.

Key Point 2: Timing Your Hydration

Don't chug water right before your workout, as it can lead to discomfort and even cramping. Instead, aim to drink fluids consistently throughout the day. About 2 hours before exercise, consume 16-20 ounces (approximately 500-600 ml) of water. Then, 10-15 minutes before your workout, have another 8-10 ounces (about 250-300 ml).

Key Point 3: Electrolytes and Rehydration

For intense workouts lasting longer than an hour, consider beverages that contain electrolytes to replenish sodium, potassium, and other essential minerals lost through sweat. Coconut water or a sports drink (preferably with no added sugars) can help with rehydration.

Mindful pre-workout nutrition involves making conscious choices about what, when, and how you eat before exercise. By fueling your body with the right balance of macros, watching your portion sizes, and timing your meals or snacks effectively, you set yourself up for success in your fitness journey. Remember that hydration is equally vital; proper fluid intake ensures you're ready to perform at your best. So, whether you're gearing up for a morning run or an afternoon yoga session, approach your pre-workout nutrition with mindfulness and intention, and watch your exercise performance soar.

10.3 Mindful Eating Post-Exercise

After the exhilarating rush of physical activity, your body is ready for rejuvenation and recovery. This is the moment when your choices about what to eat can profoundly impact your fitness journey. In this sub-chapter, we delve into the essential art of mindful eating after exercise. It's not just about refueling; it's about nourishing your body, helping it heal, and setting the stage for future successes.

Nourishing Your Body After Physical Activity

Exercise places demands on your body, depleting energy stores, and sometimes causing micro-injuries in muscles. It's during this post-exercise window that your body is most receptive to replenishment. However, what you provide matters.

1. Protein Power: After a workout, your muscles crave protein to kickstart repair and growth. Think about lean sources like chicken, tofu, beans, or a protein shake if that's your preference. Including protein-rich foods in your post-exercise meal helps rebuild muscle tissue and aids in recovery.

2. Carbohydrate Consideration: Carbohydrates are the body's primary source of energy. Post-exercise, your glycogen stores are depleted, and refilling them with healthy carbs is crucial. Opt for complex carbs like whole grains, sweet potatoes, or quinoa. They release energy slowly, helping you avoid the dreaded energy crash.

3. Hydration Hero: Don't forget about hydration. Water is your workout buddy's best friend. Sweating removes essential fluids and electrolytes, so drinking water helps maintain your body's equilibrium.

Post-Workout Recovery Foods

The perfect post-workout meal doesn't have to be complicated. In fact, simplicity often reigns supreme. Here are some easy and nourishing options:

- Grilled Chicken Salad: A lean protein source paired with leafy greens, cherry tomatoes, and a drizzle of olive oil-based dressing is a satisfying choice.

- Smoothie: Blend together some frozen berries, a banana, a scoop of plant-based protein powder, and almond milk for a quick, refreshing post-workout drink.

- Avocado Toast: Spread ripe avocado on whole-grain toast and sprinkle with a pinch of salt and red pepper flakes. It's a delightful combo of healthy fats, carbs, and protein.

- Greek Yogurt Parfait: Layer Greek yogurt with fresh fruit, honey, and a sprinkle of granola for a creamy and satisfying post-exercise treat.

- Quinoa and Veggies: Mix cooked quinoa with roasted vegetables and a drizzle of tahini dressing for a balanced and nutritious post-workout meal.

Remember, the key is to keep it balanced and tailored to your dietary preferences and restrictions. These foods offer nutrients that aid recovery and leave you feeling energized.

Listening to Your Body's Needs
Listening to your body is an art worth mastering. After exercise, your body sends signals, and understanding them is the foundation of mindful eating post-workout.

1. Hunger Signals: Pay attention to your hunger cues. Sometimes, after a strenuous workout, you might feel ravenous. In such cases, a substantial meal is in order.

Other times, your appetite may be more moderate, calling for a lighter snack.

2. Cravings vs. Necessity: It's common to crave specific foods post-exercise. Cravings often indicate your body's need for certain nutrients. For example, a craving for a banana might mean you need potassium to prevent muscle cramps.

3. Thirst Matters: Thirst can be mistaken for hunger. Ensure you're well-hydrated. If you're unsure whether you're hungry or just thirsty, try sipping water first and see if the feeling subsides.

4. Timing Is Everything: Timing is critical. Aim to eat within an hour or two after exercising when your body's recovery mechanisms are at their peak.

5. Experiment and Adapt: Every body is different. Experiment with post-workout meals and snacks to find what makes you feel your best. Whether it's a hearty breakfast or a light protein shake, personalizing your post-exercise nutrition is key.

Incorporating mindfulness into your post-exercise eating means savoring every bite, appreciating the effort you've put into your workout, and acknowledging the nourishment your body deserves.

Integrating mindful eating into your exercise routine extends beyond the gym or the yoga mat. It's a holistic approach to health that recognizes the profound connection between what you put into your body and the results you achieve.

So, as you lace up your sneakers or roll out your yoga mat, remember that what happens afterward is just as crucial. Nourish your body, respect its signals, and embrace the transformative power of mindful eating in your fitness journey. It's not just about reaching your ideal body; it's about feeling your best, inside and out.

10.4 Mindful Eating for Muscle Building

In our quest for a healthy and ideal body, it's crucial not to underestimate the profound impact of nutrition on our fitness journey. Welcome to the sub-chapter on "Mindful Eating for Muscle Building." Here, we will delve into the art of fueling your workouts with mindful nutrition, the essential role of protein in muscle recovery, and the importance of balancing macronutrients mindfully. Let's embark on this empowering and action-oriented journey to enhance your muscle-building efforts through the lens of mindfulness.

Fueling Your Workouts with Mindful Nutrition

Imagine your body as a high-performance vehicle, and the food you consume as the fuel that powers it. Just as you wouldn't expect a sports car to perform optimally on low-quality gasoline, your body needs the right nutrients to excel during workouts. Mindful eating for muscle building starts with understanding the intricacies of nutrition.

Key Point 1: Protein Powerhouse

When it comes to muscle building, protein is the unsung hero. It's the primary building block for muscles and plays a pivotal role in muscle repair and growth. As you engage in strength training and resistance exercises, you create tiny tears in your muscle fibers. Protein swoops in like a superhero to repair and rebuild these fibers, making them stronger and larger.

Mindful eating for muscle building means being intentional about your protein intake. Opt for lean sources like chicken, turkey, fish, tofu, beans, and lentils. The timing of your protein consumption matters too. To maximize muscle protein synthesis, aim to include protein-rich foods in your meals shortly after your workout. It's like giving your muscles the tools they need to rebuild and grow stronger.

Key Point 2: Carbohydrates: Your Energy Source

Carbohydrates often get a bad rap in the world of dieting, but they are your body's primary source of energy, especially during intense workouts. Complex carbohydrates, found in foods like whole grains, brown rice, quinoa, and sweet potatoes, provide a steady release of energy, helping you power through those grueling training sessions.

Mindful eating involves recognizing when your body needs that extra fuel boost. Prioritize carbohydrates in your pre-workout meals to ensure you have the energy to push your limits. It's all about balance and timing, providing your body with the energy it needs when it needs it.

Key Point 3: Healthy Fats for Recovery

While protein and carbohydrates are the stars of the muscle-building show, don't forget about healthy fats. Omega-3 fatty acids, found in fatty fish, flaxseeds, and walnuts, have anti-inflammatory properties that can aid in post-workout recovery. Inflammation is a natural response to exercise, but excessive inflammation can hinder muscle repair and growth. Mindful eating involves incorporating these healthy fats into your diet to support recovery.

In a nutshell, mindful eating for muscle building is about nourishing your body with the right nutrients at the right times. It's a strategy that empowers you to optimize your workouts, reduce the risk of injury, and accelerate muscle growth.

Protein and Muscle Recovery
Now, let's dive deeper into the incredible role that protein plays in muscle recovery. You might have heard the saying, "You are what you eat." When it comes to muscle recovery, that saying couldn't be more accurate.

The Protein Puzzle

Protein, composed of amino acids, is like the puzzle pieces that come together to rebuild and repair your muscles. When you engage in resistance training or intense exercise, you create micro-tears in your muscle fibers. Your body responds by signaling for amino acids to come to the rescue and patch up those tears. This process is known as muscle protein synthesis, and it's the foundation of muscle growth and repair.

Imagine your muscles as a construction site, with protein as the construction workers and amino acids as the building materials. The more efficiently this process occurs, the faster your muscles recover and grow.

Protein Timing

Timing matters when it comes to protein consumption. After a workout, your muscles are primed to absorb nutrients like a sponge. This is commonly referred to as the "anabolic window." During this period, which lasts for several hours post-exercise, your muscles are particularly receptive to protein.

Mindful eating for muscle recovery means capitalizing on this window of opportunity. Within a couple of hours after your workout, aim to consume a balanced meal or snack rich in protein. This could be a protein shake, a serving of Greek yogurt, or a hearty quinoa and vegetable bowl with tofu. By doing so, you enhance the muscle repair process and set the stage for growth.

Protein Quantity

How much protein do you need for optimal muscle recovery and growth? The answer varies depending on factors such as your age, sex, and activity level. As a general guideline, consider aiming for about 20-25 grams of high-quality protein in your post-workout meal or snack.

However, it's important to remember that more isn't always better. Your body can only utilize a certain amount of protein at a time. Excess protein consumption can lead to the breakdown of amino acids for energy rather than muscle repair. It's all about finding the right balance that suits your individual needs and goals.

Diversify Your Protein Sources

While protein shakes and supplements can be convenient, don't rely solely on them for your protein intake. Diversify your protein sources to ensure you receive a wide range of essential amino acids. Incorporate lean meats, poultry, fish, plant-based sources like beans and lentils, and dairy or dairy alternatives into your diet.

Remember, the path to muscle recovery and growth isn't paved with protein alone. It's a combination of nutrients, including carbohydrates, healthy fats, vitamins, and minerals, that work in harmony to support your fitness goals.

Balancing Macronutrients Mindfully
In the world of nutrition, the term "macronutrients" refers to the three primary components of your diet: carbohydrates, proteins, and fats. Each of these macronutrients plays a unique role in your body's functions,

including energy production, muscle growth, and overall health. Mindful eating for muscle building involves understanding and balancing these macronutrients mindfully.

Carbohydrates: The Energy Source

Carbohydrates, often given a bad reputation in trendy diets, are your body's primary source of energy. When you consume carbohydrates, your body breaks them down into glucose, which provides the fuel necessary for your workouts. During exercise, your muscles rely on glucose to perform optimally.

Mindful eating acknowledges the importance of carbohydrates for energy. Before a workout, especially a high-intensity one, prioritize complex carbohydrates like whole grains, legumes, and starchy vegetables. These foods release energy slowly, ensuring you have the stamina to power through your training session.

Proteins: The Muscle Builders

As discussed earlier, proteins are the building blocks of muscle. They contain amino acids, which are essential for repairing and building muscle tissue. When you engage in strength training or resistance exercises, you create tiny tears in your muscles. Proteins swoop in to mend these tears, resulting in muscle growth and increased strength.

Mindful eating emphasizes the significance of protein not only for muscle repair but also for overall health. Include lean sources of protein in your diet, such as poultry, fish, tofu, and legumes. Distribute your protein intake throughout the day, ensuring that your body has a steady supply of amino acids to support muscle growth.

Healthy Fats: The Recovery Boosters

While carbohydrates and proteins take the spotlight, healthy fats shouldn't be overlooked. Omega-3 fatty acids, found in fatty fish, flaxseeds, and walnuts, have anti-inflammatory properties that aid in post-workout recovery. Excessive inflammation can impede muscle repair and hinder your fitness progress.

Mindful eating encourages the incorporation of healthy fats into your diet to support recovery. While they don't provide energy during your workouts like carbohydrates, they play a crucial role in reducing inflammation and enhancing overall recovery.

Balancing macronutrients mindfully isn't about rigidly counting grams or following strict ratios. It's about creating a balanced and sustainable approach to nutrition that aligns with your fitness goals. Different workouts and activities may require variations in your macronutrient intake. For instance, endurance athletes may need more carbohydrates, while strength trainers may require additional protein.

To find your ideal macronutrient balance, consider seeking guidance from a registered dietitian or nutritionist. They can provide personalized recommendations based on your specific needs and goals. Remember that mindful eating isn't about restriction but rather about making informed choices that empower your fitness journey.

Mindful eating for muscle building involves understanding the role of macronutrients—carbohydrates, proteins, and fats—in optimizing your workouts and supporting muscle recovery. It's about fueling your body with intention, providing it with the right nutrients at the right times, and finding the balance that aligns with your fitness goals. When you combine mindful nutrition with regular exercise, you set the stage for a transformative journey towards a stronger, healthier you.

10.5 Mindful Eating Progress & Tracking

In our journey towards better health and our ideal bodies, we've explored the profound impact of mindful eating and exercise. We've delved into the realms of mindful consumption, the fusion of food and emotions, and the way these practices can transform our lives. But there's more to this journey than just the initial steps. This Sub-Chapter, "Mindful Eating Progress & Tracking," takes us deeper into the heart of our efforts. It's where we learn how to create a balanced and sustainable meal and exercise plan, track our progress, and ensure that mindful eating and exercise become the keystones of our long-term success.

Creating a Balanced and Sustainable Meal & Exercise Plan

One of the keys to a successful mindful eating and exercise journey is balance. It's not about extremes or quick fixes; it's about finding equilibrium in our lives. Think of it as creating a symphony where food and movement dance together in harmony.

To achieve this balance, start by setting clear, achievable goals. These goals should be specific, measurable, and realistic. Instead of saying, "I want to lose weight," try "I want to lose 10 pounds in the next three months by practicing mindful eating and exercising regularly."

Next, craft a meal plan that supports your goals. In the world of mindful eating, quality often outweighs quantity. Focus on nutrient-dense foods like whole grains, lean proteins, and an abundance of colorful fruits and vegetables. Embrace the wisdom of Mediterranean cuisine or Japanese delicacies, finding inspiration in the vibrant flavors they offer. Remember that a meal plan doesn't need to be restrictive; it should be enjoyable, sustainable, and adaptable.

Similarly, your exercise plan should be a source of inspiration, not dread. Find activities that you genuinely enjoy and that align with your goals. Whether it's yoga, dancing, hiking, or hitting the gym, make it an integral part of your routine. Consistency is key. Treat your workouts as appointments with yourself, and honor them as you would any other commitment.

Tracking Progress and Adapting Your Approach

Now that you have your balanced plan in place, it's time to start tracking your progress. Tracking isn't just about numbers on a scale or miles run; it's about assessing how you feel, both physically and emotionally.

Start a journal to record your meals, workouts, and how you felt during and after each. This journal becomes a valuable tool to identify patterns, triggers, and progress. Did you feel more energetic after a certain meal? Did a particular exercise leave you feeling invigorated or drained?

As you track your progress, be compassionate with yourself. There will be days when you indulge a bit more or skip a workout, and that's perfectly okay. Mindful eating and exercise are about nurturing your body and mind, not punishing yourself for perceived failures. Embrace these moments as opportunities to learn and grow.

When it comes to metrics, remember that progress isn't always linear. While the numbers on the scale or your fitness level are important indicators, they don't tell the whole story. Pay attention to how your clothes fit, your increased stamina, or how your mood and confidence have improved. These non-scale victories are often the most empowering.

Adaptability is another key to long-term success. Life is dynamic, and so should be your approach to mindful eating and exercise. If you find that a particular meal plan or workout routine isn't working for you, don't hesitate to

make changes. Your journey is unique, and your plan
should evolve with you.

Mindful Eating & Exercise for Long-Term Success
We've laid the foundation for mindful eating and exercise,
created a balanced plan, and tracked our progress. Now,
let's talk about the long game. It's not just about reaching
our ideal body; it's about maintaining it and thriving in our
new, healthier lifestyle.

Mindful eating and exercise are not temporary fixes; they
are lifelong practices. Think of them as your faithful
companions on the journey of life. To ensure their
permanence, make them integral parts of your daily routine.
Make them as essential as brushing your teeth or getting
dressed. When mindful eating and exercise become habits,
they cease to be chores and transform into empowering
rituals.

A key aspect of long-term success is the support system
you build around you. Share your journey with friends,
family, or a community of like-minded individuals. Their
encouragement, shared experiences, and accountability can
make all the difference. Remember, you're not alone on this
path.

Celebrate your successes, no matter how small they may
seem. Each mindful choice you make, each workout
completed, is a step closer to your ideal body and a
healthier, more fulfilling life. Treat yourself with kindness

and appreciation. Positive reinforcement can be a powerful motivator.

Integrating mindful eating with exercise is not a sprint; it's a marathon. It's a journey of self-discovery, transformation, and lasting change. Embrace balance, track your progress with compassion, and keep your eyes on the horizon of long-term success. Your ideal body is not a distant dream; it's a reality waiting for you to claim it through the empowering practice of mindful living.

Chapter 11: Mindful Eating and Personal Transformation

11.1 The Path to Holistic Mindfulness

In the quest for personal transformation, we often seek profound change in one aspect of our lives—whether it's achieving physical fitness, emotional balance, or mental clarity. However, true transformation transcends these isolated pursuits. It delves into the heart of who we are, connecting our mind, body, and spirit in a profound dance of interconnectedness. Welcome to the path of holistic mindfulness, a journey that can revolutionize your relationship with food, your body, and your very existence.

Understanding Holistic Mindfulness

Holistic mindfulness is not just a buzzword or a new-age concept. It is a profound state of awareness that integrates every facet of your being into a harmonious whole. It is a state where you perceive your thoughts, emotions, sensations, and actions as interconnected and inseparable.

To understand holistic mindfulness, imagine yourself standing at the center of a web, with each strand representing a different aspect of your existence. Your thoughts, like threads, are woven into the fabric of your emotions. Your emotions, in turn, influence the sensations in your body. Your body, through its health and vitality, impacts the energy of your spirit. This intricate web is the essence of holistic mindfulness.

At its core, holistic mindfulness means paying attention to the present moment without judgment. It involves observing your thoughts, feelings, and bodily sensations as they arise, acknowledging them without attaching labels of "good" or "bad." This non-judgmental observation allows you to gain a deeper understanding of yourself and your inner workings.

The Interconnectedness of Mind, Body, and Spirit
Now, let's explore the profound interconnectedness of your mind, body, and spirit within the context of holistic mindfulness.

Mind: Your mind is a powerful force. It generates thoughts, beliefs, and perceptions that shape your reality. When you practice mindful eating, you begin to recognize the intimate connection between your thoughts and your relationship with food. Negative self-talk, for example, can lead to emotional eating, while a positive mindset can inspire healthier choices.

But it doesn't stop there. Your thoughts also affect your emotions. When you harbor stress-inducing thoughts about food or body image, your emotional state becomes tense. This emotional turmoil, in turn, manifests as physical sensations like muscle tension or a racing heart. Your mind's power over your body is undeniable.

Body: Your body is a living, breathing manifestation of your inner world. It responds to your thoughts and emotions with astonishing precision. Think about the last time you felt anxious—your heart rate increased, your muscles tightened, and your breath quickened. This immediate physical response to your emotional state is a testament to the mind-body connection.

When it comes to mindful eating, this connection is particularly evident. The sensations of hunger and fullness are your body's way of communicating with you. When you pay close attention to these cues without judgment, you learn to trust your body's wisdom. In contrast, ignoring these signals can lead to overeating or undereating, disrupting the delicate balance of your well-being.

Spirit: Your spirit, often considered the core of your being, is the source of your inner strength and resilience. It's where your values, purpose, and sense of self reside. Your spirit is not separate from your mind and body; rather, it's the radiant thread that weaves through the fabric of your existence.

In the context of holistic mindfulness, your spirit plays a pivotal role in your relationship with food and personal transformation. It's the wellspring of your motivation and determination to make positive changes in your life. When your spirit is aligned with your mindful eating journey, you tap into a well of inner wisdom and strength. You become the architect of your transformation, driven by a deeper sense of purpose.

Embracing a Holistic Approach to Well-being

Now that you understand the interconnectedness of your mind, body, and spirit, it's time to embrace a holistic approach to well-being. This approach is not limited to mindful eating; it encompasses all aspects of your life. Here's how you can apply holistic mindfulness to your journey of personal transformation:

1. Cultivate Self-Awareness: Begin by observing your thoughts, emotions, and bodily sensations without judgment. Notice how they influence each other. When you recognize a negative thought pattern, gently redirect it toward a more positive and empowering perspective. This self-awareness is the cornerstone of holistic mindfulness.

2. Embrace Mindful Eating: Extend your self-awareness to your relationship with food. Pay close attention to the sensations of hunger and fullness. Recognize how your emotions and thoughts impact your eating habits. By doing so, you'll develop a healthier and more intuitive approach to nourishing your body.

3. Align with Your Values: Connect with your inner values and sense of purpose. What drives your desire for personal transformation? Is it a commitment to health, vitality, or inner peace? When your goals align with your values, you'll find the motivation and perseverance to overcome challenges.

4. Practice Self-Compassion: Treat yourself with kindness and compassion. Understand that personal transformation is a journey, and there will be setbacks along the way. Instead of self-criticism, offer yourself encouragement and

understanding. This self-compassion fuels your resilience and growth.

5. Seek Balance: Balance is the essence of holistic mindfulness. Strive for balance in your thoughts, emotions, and actions. Balance the foods you eat, the exercise you engage in, and the rest you allow yourself. Balance your inner world with your outer world, and you'll find harmony in your transformation.

6. Connect with Others: Recognize that your journey of personal transformation is not isolated. Your interconnectedness extends to the people around you. Seek support from a community of like-minded individuals who share your goals. Share your experiences, learn from others, and draw strength from the collective wisdom.

Incorporating these principles of holistic mindfulness into your life is a profound step toward personal transformation. It's not just about changing your habits; it's about changing your perspective and embracing the interconnectedness of your mind, body, and spirit. This holistic approach empowers you to create lasting, meaningful change in your life, including your relationship with food and your journey toward well-being.

So, as you continue your path of personal transformation through mindful eating, remember that you are embarking on a holistic journey—a journey that honors the profound connection between your mind, body, and spirit. Embrace this connection, nurture it, and watch as it transforms not

only your eating habits but your entire existence. You have
the power to awaken the holistic mindfulness within you
and unlock the doors to personal transformation that you've
always desired. Your journey has just begun, and the
possibilities are limitless.

11.2 Mindful Eating as a Gateway to Holistic Living

In the journey of personal transformation, we often seek
profound change that extends beyond surface-level
alterations. We yearn for a shift in consciousness, a deeper
connection to ourselves and the world around us. It's within
this context that mindful eating emerges as a gateway to
holistic living, offering a path to profound personal
transformation.

The Practice of Mindful Eating as Mindfulness in Action

Mindfulness, in its essence, is the practice of being fully
present in the moment, without judgment or distraction. It's
about acknowledging our experiences as they unfold and
embracing them with an open heart. Mindful eating is not
an exception; it's mindfulness in action. When we engage
in this practice, we bring our full attention to the act of
eating, savoring each bite as if it were our first and last.

Imagine sitting down to a meal, and instead of wolfing
down your food while watching TV or scrolling through

your smartphone, you savor every morsel. You notice the vibrant colors of your plate, the aroma that dances through the air, and the textures that play on your taste buds. With each bite, you appreciate the journey the food took to reach your plate – the sun, the soil, the hands that nurtured it. This is mindfulness in action, my friends.

As you embark on this journey of mindful eating, you'll begin to notice the subtle shifts in your relationship with food. You'll become more attuned to your body's hunger and fullness cues. You'll discern between physical hunger and emotional hunger, and you'll find that the latter often dissipates with mindfulness. Your cravings will lose their grip on you, and you'll gain a newfound sense of control over your eating choices.

How Mindful Eating Extends Beyond the Plate
Now, let's talk about the magic of mindful eating, which extends far beyond the boundaries of your dinner plate. When you engage in this practice consistently, you'll find that it permeates every aspect of your life. You'll become more conscious of the choices you make – not just about food, but about how you spend your time, who you surround yourself with, and how you nourish your mind and soul.

The mindfulness cultivated through mindful eating seeps into your daily routines. You begin to appreciate the small moments – the warm rays of sunshine on your skin, the laughter of a loved one, the rustle of leaves in the wind.

Each moment becomes an opportunity for mindfulness, a chance to fully immerse yourself in the richness of life.

In your interactions with others, you'll find yourself more present, more attuned to their words and feelings. You'll listen not just with your ears but with your heart, offering your full attention and empathy. Relationships flourish under the care of a mindful heart.

Cultivating Awareness in All Aspects of Life
Now, let's delve into the heart of the matter – how mindful eating can serve as a catalyst for personal transformation. When you approach each meal with intention and presence, it becomes a mirror reflecting your relationship with yourself and the world around you.

As you savor the flavors and textures of your food, you become intimately acquainted with your body's signals. You recognize when you're truly hungry and when you're simply seeking comfort or distraction. This heightened self-awareness spills over into other areas of your life.

You may find yourself asking questions like, "Am I truly fulfilled by my job?" or "Am I living in alignment with my values and aspirations?" The same mindfulness that guided you to choose nourishing foods can guide you toward making choices that align with your deeper purpose.

Beyond the physical and emotional benefits, mindful eating can help you cultivate a sense of gratitude for the abundance in your life. It's not just about appreciating the food on your plate; it's about recognizing the abundance of experiences, relationships, and opportunities that surround you. Gratitude, after all, is the foundation of lasting joy and contentment.

As you continue on your journey of mindful eating, you may notice that you become more attuned to the natural rhythms of life. You'll awaken to the changing seasons, the cycles of the moon, and the beauty of the present moment. This heightened awareness can lead to a deeper sense of connection with the world and a profound shift in your perspective.

So, my dear readers, as you embrace mindful eating as a gateway to holistic living, remember that it's not just about the act of eating; it's about the art of living. It's about savoring every moment, finding purpose in each choice, and awakening to the profound beauty of the world around you. Mindful eating is the first step on a transformative journey – a journey toward a more conscious, meaningful, and joyful life.

11.3 Mindful Living Beyond Food

In your journey toward personal transformation through mindful eating, it's essential to understand that mindfulness extends far beyond what you put on your plate. While conscious eating is a potent catalyst for change, the practice of mindfulness can profoundly impact various aspects of your life. In this sub-chapter, we'll explore how to apply mindfulness to different areas of your existence, from time management to finding joy in the mundane.

Applying Mindfulness to Various Aspects of Life
Mindfulness is a way of living, not just a mealtime ritual. It's about paying unwavering attention to the present moment in all that you do. Whether you're at work, spending time with loved ones, or engaged in solitary activities, mindfulness can be your steadfast companion.

When you approach daily tasks with mindfulness, you cultivate a heightened awareness that can lead to personal growth and transformation. Here are a few ways to weave mindfulness into your daily life:

- Mindful Communication: Mindful eating begins with understanding your relationship with food. Similarly, mindful communication starts with understanding your relationship with words. Take time to listen actively, speak intentionally, and communicate with empathy. By doing so, you can foster deeper connections and more meaningful relationships.

- Mindful Work: Apply mindfulness to your professional life by practicing present-moment awareness. It can enhance your productivity, creativity, and job satisfaction. Engage fully in your work, whether it's a complex project or routine tasks. By focusing on one task at a time and giving it your full attention, you can accomplish more and experience a sense of achievement.

- Mindful Relationships: Interactions with others are a crucial aspect of life. When you're fully present in your relationships, you can build deeper connections and resolve conflicts more effectively. Mindful listening and empathetic responses can transform your interactions, making them more authentic and fulfilling.

Mindful Time Management and Productivity
Time is a finite resource, and how you manage it can significantly impact your personal transformation journey. Mindful time management isn't about cramming more into your schedule but rather about making conscious choices about how you spend your time.

Here are some practical steps to incorporate mindful time management into your life:

- Prioritize with Purpose: Mindful time management begins with setting clear priorities. Ask yourself what truly matters to you and align your activities with your values and goals. Eliminate tasks that don't contribute to your well-being or personal growth.

- Single-Tasking: In a world that often celebrates multitasking, the art of single-tasking is a form of mindfulness. Focus on one task at a time, giving it your full attention and energy. This approach not only boosts productivity but also allows you to savor the process.

- Mindful Scheduling: Create a schedule that allows for mindful transitions between activities. Give yourself buffer time to decompress between meetings or tasks. Use this time to breathe, reflect, or engage in a quick mindfulness practice to reset and refocus.

- Technology Boundaries: Mindful time management also involves setting boundaries with technology. Constant notifications and digital distractions can fragment your attention. Designate specific times for checking emails or social media, and disconnect during your mindful moments.

Finding Joy and Fulfillment in Everyday Moments
Often, personal transformation is thought to be a grand and sweeping journey. However, it's the accumulation of small, mindful moments that can lead to lasting change. Finding joy and fulfillment in the seemingly mundane aspects of life is a powerful tool for personal growth.

Here's how you can infuse everyday moments with mindfulness:

- Morning Rituals: Start your day with intention and mindfulness. Whether it's savoring your morning coffee or taking a few moments of silence, create a morning ritual that sets a positive tone for the day ahead.

- Mindful Nature Connection: Spending time in nature can be a profound source of joy and rejuvenation. Mindfully observe the beauty of the natural world, whether it's the rustling of leaves in the wind or the colors of a sunset.

- Gratitude Practice: Cultivate gratitude by regularly reflecting on the things you appreciate in life. Gratitude can shift your focus from what's lacking to what's abundant, fostering a sense of fulfillment.

- Mindful Creativity: Engage in creative activities like art, writing, or music with mindfulness. The process of creation itself can be a form of meditation, allowing you to express yourself authentically and find joy in the act of creating.

Incorporating mindfulness into various aspects of your life isn't just about enhancing your personal transformation journey; it's about living a more meaningful and fulfilling existence. It's about cherishing each moment, whether ordinary or extraordinary, and recognizing that every experience has the potential to contribute to your growth and well-being.

As you continue your mindful eating practice and extend mindfulness to every facet of your life, you'll discover that personal transformation isn't a destination but a lifelong journey. Each moment is an opportunity for growth, and mindfulness is your trusted guide on this path toward a more fulfilling, purposeful, and authentic life. So, take each step with intention, and may your journey be one of continuous self-discovery and transformation.

Bonus Chapter : Example of Mindful Eating & Exercise Plan

Example 1
Morning: Mindful Breakfast

- Meal:

  - A bowl of oatmeal topped with fresh berries, a drizzle of honey, and a sprinkle of chopped nuts.

  - A side of Greek yogurt with a dash of cinnamon.

  - A glass of water or herbal tea.

- Mindful Eating Practices:

  - Sit down at a table free from distractions.

  - Take a few deep breaths before starting.

  - Chew each bite slowly and savor the flavors.

  - Pay attention to the texture and temperature of your food.

  - Pause between bites to check in with your hunger and fullness cues.

  - Stop eating when you feel satisfied, not overly full.

Exercise: Morning Yoga

- Routine: 20-30 minutes of gentle yoga poses, focusing on deep, mindful breathing and gentle stretches.

- Mindful Exercise Practices:

  - Concentrate on your breath, inhaling deeply through your nose and exhaling slowly through your mouth.

  - Pay attention to the sensations in your body as you move through each yoga pose.

  - Stay present in the moment, letting go of distracting thoughts.

  - Use yoga as a time to center yourself and set positive intentions for the day.

Lunch: Mindful Midday Meal

- Meal:

  - Grilled chicken breast with a side of steamed broccoli and quinoa.

  - A mixed greens salad with a homemade vinaigrette dressing.

  - A glass of water or herbal tea.

- Mindful Eating Practices:

- Eat slowly and savor the flavors of each component of your meal.

  - Put your fork down between bites to avoid rushing.

  - Listen to your body's hunger and fullness signals.

  - Reflect on the nourishment each bite provides.

Afternoon: Mindful Snack

- Snack:

  - A small handful of mixed nuts and dried fruits.

  - A piece of dark chocolate.

  - A glass of water or herbal tea.

- Mindful Eating Practices:

  - Choose a quiet space to enjoy your snack.

  - Pay attention to the crunch and taste of the nuts and the sweetness of the fruits.

  - Savor the chocolate slowly and mindfully.

  - Pause and take a few breaths between bites.

Exercise: Afternoon Walk

- Routine: A 30-minute brisk walk in a natural setting, such as a park.

- Mindful Exercise Practices:

  - Observe the beauty of nature around you.

  - Focus on your breath and the rhythm of your steps.

  - Let go of stress and worries, allowing the walk to clear your mind.

Dinner: Mindful Evening Meal

- Meal:

  - Baked salmon with lemon and herbs.

  - Steamed asparagus and brown rice.

  - A side of mixed greens with a light balsamic vinaigrette.

  - A glass of water or herbal tea.

- Mindful Eating Practices:

  - Set a pleasant atmosphere for dinner with dimmed lighting and soothing music.

  - Eat slowly and deliberately, savoring the flavors of your meal.

- Reflect on the nutritional value and benefits of your food.

- Stop eating when you feel comfortably satisfied.

Evening: Mindful Reflection

- Take a few minutes to reflect on your day, expressing gratitude for the nourishment and movement your body received.

- Practice a short mindfulness meditation to relax and prepare for a restful night's sleep.

Remember that this is just one example of a mindful eating meal and exercise plan. You can tailor it to your individual preferences and dietary needs. The key is to approach each meal and exercise session with mindfulness, paying attention to your body's signals and fully engaging in the present moment.

Example 2: Vegan Based

Morning: Mindful Vegan Breakfast

- Meal:

  - Vegan overnight oats made with rolled oats, almond milk, chia seeds, and topped with fresh berries, sliced bananas, and a drizzle of maple syrup.

  - A glass of freshly squeezed orange juice.

- Mindful Eating Practices:

  - Sit down at a table free from distractions.

  - Take a few deep breaths before starting.

  - Chew each bite slowly and savor the flavors.

  - Pay attention to the texture and temperature of your food.

  - Pause between bites to check in with your hunger and fullness cues.

  - Stop eating when you feel satisfied, not overly full.

Exercise: Morning Vegan Yoga

- Routine: 20-30 minutes of gentle yoga poses, focusing on deep, mindful breathing and gentle stretches.

- Mindful Exercise Practices:

  - Concentrate on your breath, inhaling deeply through your nose and exhaling slowly through your mouth.

  - Pay attention to the sensations in your body as you move through each yoga pose.

  - Stay present in the moment, letting go of distracting thoughts.

  - Use yoga as a time to center yourself and set positive intentions for the day.

Lunch: Mindful Vegan Midday Meal

- Meal:

  - Vegan Buddha bowl with quinoa, roasted chickpeas, sautéed kale, shredded carrots, and a tahini dressing.

  - A glass of lemon-infused water.

- Mindful Eating Practices:

  - Eat slowly and savor the flavors of each component of your meal.

  - Put your fork down between bites to avoid rushing.

  - Listen to your body's hunger and fullness signals.

  - Reflect on the nourishment each bite provides.

Afternoon: Mindful Vegan Snack

- Snack:

  - Sliced cucumber and bell pepper with homemade hummus.

  - A piece of fruit (e.g., apple or pear).

  - A glass of herbal tea.

- Mindful Eating Practices:

  - Choose a quiet space to enjoy your snack.

  - Pay attention to the crunch and taste of the veggies and the creaminess of the hummus.

  - Savor the fruit slowly and mindfully.

  - Pause and take a few breaths between bites.

Exercise: Afternoon Vegan Nature Walk

- Routine: A 30-minute brisk walk in a natural setting, such as a park or forest.

- Mindful Exercise Practices:

  - Observe the beauty of nature around you.

  - Focus on your breath and the rhythm of your steps.

- Let go of stress and worries, allowing the walk to clear your mind.

Dinner: Mindful Vegan Evening Meal

- Meal:

  - Vegan lentil and vegetable stew with a side of whole-grain bread.

  - Steamed broccoli with a sprinkle of nutritional yeast.

  - A glass of herbal tea.

- Mindful Eating Practices:

  - Set a pleasant atmosphere for dinner with dimmed lighting and soothing music.

  - Eat slowly and deliberately, savoring the flavors of your meal.

  - Reflect on the nutritional value and benefits of your food.

  - Stop eating when you feel comfortably satisfied.

Evening: Mindful Reflection

- Take a few minutes to reflect on your day, expressing gratitude for the nourishment and movement your body received.

- Practice a short mindfulness meditation to relax and prepare for a restful night's sleep.

This vegan mindful eating meal and exercise plan provides a balanced and nourishing day while focusing on plant-based options. Adjust the meals and exercises according to your preferences and dietary needs, all while approaching each moment with mindfulness and intention.

Example 3: Mediterranean-inspired

Morning: Mindful Mediterranean Breakfast

- Meal:

  - A Mediterranean-inspired tofu scramble with diced tomatoes, spinach, olives, and a sprinkle of oregano and nutritional yeast.

  - A side of whole-grain toast drizzled with extra virgin olive oil.

  - A serving of fresh fruit salad (e.g., citrus fruits, melon, and berries).

  - A cup of herbal tea or black coffee (if desired).

- Mindful Eating Practices:

  - Sit down at a table free from distractions.

  - Take a few deep breaths before starting.

  - Chew each bite slowly and savor the flavors.

  - Pay attention to the texture and temperature of your food.

  - Pause between bites to check in with your hunger and fullness cues.

  - Stop eating when you feel satisfied, not overly full.

Exercise: Morning Mediterranean Yoga

- Routine: 20-30 minutes of gentle yoga poses, incorporating deep, mindful breathing and stretches inspired by the Mediterranean way of life.

- Mindful Exercise Practices:

  - Visualize yourself in a serene Mediterranean coastal setting.

  - Concentrate on your breath, inhaling the fresh sea breeze and exhaling stress.

  - Incorporate flowing movements that mimic the calm waves of the Mediterranean Sea.

  - Use yoga as a time to connect with nature and cultivate a sense of tranquility.

Lunch: Mindful Mediterranean Midday Meal

- Meal:

  - Mediterranean quinoa salad with cucumber, cherry tomatoes, red onion, Kalamata olives, fresh parsley, and a lemon-olive oil dressing.

  - A serving of hummus with whole-grain pita bread.

  - A glass of cucumber-infused water.

- Mindful Eating Practices:

  - Eat slowly and savor the flavors of each component of your meal.

  - Put your fork down between bites to avoid rushing.

  - Listen to your body's hunger and fullness signals.

  - Reflect on the vibrant colors and Mediterranean flavors of your food.

Afternoon: Mindful Mediterranean Snack

- Snack:

  - A small bowl of mixed nuts (e.g., almonds, walnuts, and pistachios).

  - Sliced cucumber and carrot sticks with tzatziki sauce.

  - A glass of mint tea.

- Mindful Eating Practices:

  - Choose a quiet space to enjoy your snack.

  - Pay attention to the crunch and taste of the nuts and the coolness of the veggies.

  - Savor each bite mindfully.

  - Pause and take a few breaths between bites.

Exercise: Afternoon Mediterranean Walk

- Routine: A 30-minute leisurely walk along a scenic path or waterfront, visualizing the beauty of the Mediterranean coast.

- Mindful Exercise Practices:

  - Imagine the sound of waves crashing on the shore as you walk.

  - Focus on your breath and the sensation of your feet meeting the ground.

  - Use this walk to embrace the Mediterranean lifestyle of relaxation and appreciation for nature.

Dinner: Mindful Mediterranean Evening Meal

- Meal:

  - Grilled Mediterranean vegetables (e.g., eggplant, zucchini, and bell peppers) with a balsamic glaze.

  - Mediterranean-style lentil soup with lemon and cumin.

  - A serving of tabbouleh salad with bulgur wheat, fresh herbs, diced cucumbers, and tomatoes.

  - A glass of red wine or sparkling water with a twist of lemon (if desired).

- Mindful Eating Practices:

  - Set a pleasant atmosphere for dinner with soft lighting and Mediterranean music.

  - Eat slowly and deliberately, savoring the flavors of your meal.

  - Reflect on the health benefits and rich history of Mediterranean cuisine.

  - Stop eating when you feel comfortably satisfied.

Evening: Mindful Reflection

- Take a few minutes to reflect on your day, appreciating the Mediterranean-inspired flavors and the peaceful moments you experienced.

- Practice a short mindfulness meditation to relax and prepare for a restful night's sleep.

This Mediterranean-inspired mindful eating meal and exercise plan combines the healthful aspects of Mediterranean cuisine with mindfulness practices for a balanced and enjoyable day. As always, adjust the meals and exercises to suit your preferences and dietary needs while approaching each moment with mindfulness and gratitude.

Example 4: Japanese Cuisine

Morning: Mindful Japanese Breakfast

- Meal:

  - A traditional Japanese breakfast featuring miso soup with tofu and seaweed.

  - Steamed rice topped with a poached egg and pickled vegetables (tsukemono).

  - A side of grilled fish (or a vegan alternative like grilled tempeh).

  - Green tea (matcha or sencha) with a small sweet treat like a red bean paste mochi.

- Mindful Eating Practices:

  - Sit down at a low table or on a cushion, embracing the Japanese dining style.

  - Begin with a moment of gratitude (itadakimasu).

  - Use chopsticks mindfully, paying attention to each bite.

  - Sip the green tea slowly, appreciating its soothing warmth.

  - Reflect on the balance and variety of flavors in your meal.

Exercise: Morning Japanese Tai Chi

- Routine: 20-30 minutes of gentle Tai Chi movements inspired by the serenity of Japanese gardens.

- Mindful Exercise Practices:

  - Visualize yourself in a tranquil Japanese garden, surrounded by nature.

  - Focus on slow, flowing movements and deep, rhythmic breathing.

  - Use Tai Chi as a time to cultivate inner calm and balance.

Lunch: Mindful Japanese Midday Meal

- Meal:

  - Bento box with a variety of components: sushi rolls, tempura vegetables, edamame, and a small salad.

  - A bowl of clear miso soup with green onions and seaweed.

  - A serving of fresh fruit (e.g., sliced oranges or persimmons).

- Mindful Eating Practices:

- Open your bento box with anticipation and appreciation for the presentation.

 - Savor each bite of sushi, tempura, and salad.

 - Enjoy the miso soup as a comforting and nourishing element of your meal.

 - Reflect on the harmony of flavors and textures in your bento.

Afternoon: Mindful Japanese Snack

- Snack:

 - A plate of sliced cucumbers and carrots with a dollop of sesame miso dip.

 - A cup of hojicha (roasted green tea) or genmaicha (green tea with roasted rice).

- Mindful Eating Practices:

 - Choose a quiet space to enjoy your snack.

 - Pay attention to the crispness of the vegetables and the umami richness of the dip.

 - Savor each bite slowly and mindfully.

 - Pause and take a few breaths between bites.

Exercise: Afternoon Japanese Nature Walk

- Routine: A 30-minute walk in a serene natural setting, imagining the tranquility of a Japanese forest.

- Mindful Exercise Practices:

  - Visualize yourself strolling through a peaceful Japanese forest.

  - Focus on your breath and the rhythm of your steps.

  - Let go of stress and tension, embracing the calming influence of nature.

Dinner: Mindful Japanese Evening Meal

- Meal:

  - Nabe hot pot with a variety of vegetables, tofu, and thinly sliced shiitake mushrooms in a savory broth.

  - A bowl of white or brown rice.

  - A side of sunomono (cucumber salad) with a light rice vinegar dressing.

  - A glass of cold green tea (sencha or gyokuro).

- Mindful Eating Practices:

  - Set a peaceful atmosphere for dinner with minimal lighting.

- Carefully add ingredients to the hot pot and enjoy the communal experience.

- Savor the flavors of the simmering hot pot and the simplicity of the rice.

- Reflect on the balance and nourishment of your meal.

Evening: Mindful Reflection

- Take a few minutes to reflect on your day, appreciating the Japanese-inspired flavors and mindfulness moments.

- Practice a short mindfulness meditation to relax and prepare for a restful night's sleep.

This Japanese-inspired mindful eating meal and exercise plan incorporates the flavors and traditions of Japanese cuisine into a day of mindfulness. Feel free to adapt the meals and exercises to suit your preferences and dietary needs while savoring each moment with gratitude and mindfulness.

Conclusion

Congratulations on reaching the end of this transformative journey! You've embarked on a path of self-discovery, mindful eating, and personal growth. As we close the chapters of this book, it's not the end but rather a new beginning for you.

Throughout this book, we've delved into the profound impact that mindful eating can have on your life. You've learned to savor the flavors, nourish your body, and listen to your inner wisdom. But remember, mindful eating is not just a practice; it's a way of life. The journey continues beyond these pages, and the possibilities are boundless.

Crafting Your Personal Mindful Eating Plan

As you stand at the crossroads of your mindful eating journey, it's time to create a roadmap for your future. Crafting a personal mindful eating plan is your first step. Here's how you can approach it:

Setting Mindful Eating Goals: Start by defining your mindful eating goals. What specific changes do you want to make in your relationship with food and eating? Your goals might include eating more mindfully, improving your relationship with your body, or making healthier food choices.

Creating a Mindful Eating Schedule: Establish a mindful eating schedule that aligns with your daily life. Consider when and where you'll practice mindful eating. Will you incorporate it into every meal, or start with a few key moments each day?

Tracking Progress and Adjusting Your Plan: Keep a journal to track your mindful eating journey. Record your observations, challenges, and successes. Regularly review your journal to identify patterns and areas for improvement. Remember that your plan is not set in stone; it's a flexible guide that can evolve as you grow.

Staying Accountable and Motivated

Accountability is a powerful force in your mindful eating journey. It helps you stay on track and motivated. Here are some strategies to stay accountable:

Find an Accountability Partner or Group: Share your mindful eating journey with a friend, family member, or a supportive community. Having someone to check in with can provide encouragement and accountability.

Mindful Eating Check-Ins: Schedule regular check-ins with yourself to reflect on your progress. Ask yourself how you've been doing with your mindful eating goals, what challenges you've encountered, and what adjustments you can make.

Revisiting Your Ideal Body Vision

Throughout this journey, you've been guided by the vision of your ideal body. Now is the time to revisit and refine that vision. Remember that your ideal body is not a fixed image but a dynamic concept that can evolve. It's about feeling your best, nourishing your body, and embracing your uniqueness.

Mindful Eating and Self-Compassion

As you continue your mindful eating journey, it's crucial to embrace self-compassion. Be kind to yourself, especially when faced with challenges or setbacks. Remember that mindful eating is a practice, not perfection. Here's how you can cultivate self-compassion:

Embracing Self-Love and Acceptance: Practice self-love by treating yourself with the same kindness and understanding you would offer to a dear friend. Accept your body and yourself as you are right now, knowing that you are worthy of love and care.

Mindful Eating as Self-Care: View mindful eating as an act of self-care. Nourish your body with foods that make you feel good, and prioritize self-care activities that support your well-being.

Your Ongoing Journey to Your Ideal Body

In closing, remember that your mindful eating journey is not a destination; it's a lifelong path. Each day presents new opportunities for growth, self-discovery, and transformation. As you continue on this journey, keep the following principles in mind:

Consistency: Consistency is the key to lasting change. Continuously practice mindful eating, even when faced with challenges. Over time, it will become second nature.

Flexibility: Be flexible and adaptable in your approach. Your mindful eating plan can evolve as your needs and circumstances change.

Patience: Personal transformation takes time. Be patient with yourself, and acknowledge that progress may come in waves. Celebrate the journey, not just the destination.

Gratitude: Cultivate gratitude for the gift of mindfulness and the opportunity to nourish your body and soul. Gratitude can be a powerful motivator and a source of inner peace.

As you step into your future, may your mindful eating journey be a source of empowerment, self-love, and personal growth. Embrace the practice of mindful eating as a lifelong companion, guiding you toward a healthier, more fulfilling, and more authentic life. Your ideal body is not a distant dream; it is a reflection of the mindful choices you make each day. Keep walking this path with intention, and may it lead you to a life of abundance, well-being, and joy.